Development and Aging in the Nervous System

ACADEMIC PRESS RAPID MANUSCRIPT REPRODUCTION

Proceedings of a Symposium on the
Development and Aging in the Nervous System
Held in Miami, Florida
February 19-20, 1973

Development and Aging in the Nervous System

Edited by
Morris Rockstein

Associate Editor
Marvin L. Sussman

Department of Physiology and Biophysics
University of Miami School of Medicine
Miami, Florida

ACADEMIC PRESS, INC. New York and London 1973
A Subsidiary of Harcourt Brace Jovanovich, Publishers

ACADEMIC PRESS, INC.
111 Fifth Avenue, New York, New York 10003

United Kingdom Edition published by
ACADEMIC PRESS, INC. (LONDON) LTD.
24/28 Oval Road, London NW1

Library of Congress Cataloging in Publication Data

Symposium on the Development and Aging in the Nervous System, Miami, Fla., 1973.

Development and aging in the nervous system.

1. Nervous system–Aging–Congresses. 2. Developmental neurology–Congresses. I. Rockstein, Morris, ed. II. Title. [DNLM: 1. Aging–Congresses. 2. Nervous system–Growth and development–Congresses. WL102 S9825d 1973]
QP356.S94 1973 612'.8 73-2081
ISBN 0–12–591650–7

PRINTED IN THE UNITED STATES OF AMERICA

CONTENTS

CONTRIBUTORS

William Bondareff, Department of Anatomy, Northwestern University Medical School, Chicago, Illinois 60611

Harold Brody, Department of Anatomical Sciences, State University of New York at Buffalo, Buffalo, New York 14214

W. Maxwell Cowan, Department of Anatomy, Washington University School of Medicine, St. Louis, Missouri 63110

Jean de Vellis, Laboratory of Nuclear Medicine and Radiation Biology, Department of Anatomy and Retardation Center, University of California School of Medicine, Los Angeles, California 90024

John C. Eccles, Departments of Physiology and Biophysics, State University of New York at Buffalo, School of Medicine, Buffalo, New York 14214

Caleb E. Finch, The Laboratory of Neurobiology, The Ethel Percy Andrus Gerontology Center, University of Southern California, Los Angeles, California 90007

Donald H. Ford, Department of Anatomy, State University of New York, Downstate Medical Center, Brooklyn, New York 11203

Williamina A. Himwich, Nebraska Psychiatric Institute, Omaha, Nebraska 68105

Marcus Jacobson,* Department of Biophysics, The Johns Hopkins University, Baltimore, Maryland 21218

Kalidas Nandy, Department of Anatomy, Emory University, Atlanta, Georgia 30322

Frederick Richardson, University of Miami School of Medicine, Miami, Florida 33152

*Present Address: Department of Physiology and Biophysics, University of Miami School of Medicine, Miami, Florida 33152

PREFACE

This, the third publication of the proceedings of a series of symposia, held as part of the formal graduate level course work of the University of Miami Training Program in Cellular Aging, includes the papers presented by the participants in the Symposium on "Development and Aging in the Nervous System," held on February 19 and 20, 1973, in Miami, Florida.

The subject matter of this symposium is of special interest in view of the fact that the nervous system represents one of the two major organ systems, the cells of which are incapable of replacement, i.e., are postmitotic. Equally important is the recognition that the nervous system, both directly and indirectly, is concerned with regulation not only of motor activity, in the case of skeletal muscle, but equally so as regards regulation of the functioning of the heart and the blood vessels of the circulatory system, as well as all visceral smooth muscle, via the autonomic nervous system. Moreover, through its indirect endocrine function (i.e., in the release of epinephrine and norepinephrine), the last-mentioned represents a dramatically controlling element as regards virtually all visceral functions of the body.

In the above connection, aside from the recognized age-dependent degradatory changes which occur in the skin and in skeletal muscle with advancing age, the most striking "downhill" course with advancing time, both as regards structure and function, is seen in the sensory as well as motor functions of the human organism, which are directly related to changes in cell number with the passage of time.

Accordingly, the proceedings of this symposium have special significance in considering aging in its total sense, from embryonic development through senescence of a vital organ system of the body, both whose course as well as direction can be predicted for any species, with reasonable accuracy.

As regards the participants in this symposium, the Editor is proud to present this verbatim report of the symposium proceedings, in acknowledging the participation of speakers of the highest level of competency, representing a wide range of interests in neurobiology, including anatomy, morphology, embryology, enzymology and, including the clinical implications of age as a parameter in relation to normal and pathological functioning of the nervous system.

To Professor Eccles and Professor Richardson, as well as to the Chairman of the Department of Physiology and Biophysics, Professor Werner R. Loewenstein, go special thanks by the Editor for their valuable suggestions in the early organization of the program and in obtaining the participation of a number of the symposium speakers.

The Editor owes special thanks to Mrs. Estella Cooney for her careful attention to details in insuring the accuracy and clarity of the final published version of these proceedings and in the typing of the camera copy for its publication. To his Associate Editor, Marvin L. Sussman, go the expression of the Editor's profound appreciation for his continued, tireless efforts in the joint editing of the manuscripts from their draft form to the final camera copy from which this published work has been produced.

The Training Program must express its gratitude particularly to Mead Johnson & Company Research Center and the Pharmaceuticals Division of CIBA-GEIGY Corporation, whose contributions have helped make possible both this conference as well as the publication of its proceedings.

The symposium from which this publication has resulted was supported for the most part by funds from the National Institute of Child Health and Human Development (Training Program in Cellular Aging Grant No. HD-00142), and in part by the University of Miami Department of Physiology and Biophysics.

Miami, Florida, 1973 — Morris Rockstein, Ph. D.

Development and Aging in the Nervous System

AGE CHANGES IN THE NEURONAL MICROENVIRONMENT

William Bondareff

Department of Anatomy
Northwestern University Medical School
Chicago, Illinois

The microenvironment of neurons in the brain is in large part composed of extracellular space formed by submicroscopic channels between the cellular elements (Schmitt and Samson, 1969). These channels, which include synaptic clefts, are believed to be sites of physiologically important reactions involving metabolites and ions, which support neuronal metabolism. They are little understood, especially in the mammalian central nervous system.

The properties of the brain extracellular space are relatively uninvestigated during the course of normal development and senescence. In the adult brain, a chloride space of about 25% has been determined (Koch and Woodbury, 1960), and experimental evidence indicates that Cl^- is largely extracellular (Van Harreveld *et al.*, 1966). An extracellular space of this magnitude, which is consistent with that estimated from impedence measurements (Van Harreveld, 1966), is considerably greater than the 5% space indicated by thiocyanate (Streicher, 1961), sulfate (Woodbury, 1958), and sucrose analyses (Reed and Woodbury, 1960) and demonstrated in electron micrographs of chemically-fixed nervous tissue (Horstmann and Meves, 1959). Chemical fixation is believed to cause a relative asphyxia with a concomitant intracellular relocation of extracellular water (Van Harreveld *et al.*, 1965). The distribution of intracellular and extracellular water in normal nervous tissue appears to be preserved accurately by rapid freezing, followed by gradual substitution of frozen tissue water with acetone (Van Harreveld, 1966; Malhotra and Van Harreveld, 1966). It is assumed that subsequent embedding of this substituted tissue in an epoxy resin does not significantly distort the submicroscopic distribution of tissue water.

In the cerebral cortices of young adult and immature Sprague-Dawley rats, 10, 14 and 21 days of age, we have estimated the volume of tissue occupied by extracellular space and have attempted to relate sequential volume changes during normal postnatal maturation with the onset of functional maturity (Bondareff and Pysh, 1968). The cerebral cortices were rapidly frozen in situ and the frozen tissue water substituted at -78° C with a 1% solution of osmium tetroxide in acetone. In random electron micrographs of each animal, each representing 42 μ^2 of cerebral cortical molecular layer, the volume of extracellular space was estimated stereologically (Weibel et al., 1966). In 10-day-old animals an extracellular space of 40.5% was found (Fig. 1). This diminished progressively to 31.8% at 14 days and during the third week of postnatal life, when electroencephalographic activity acquires adult-like properties (Bures, 1957; Deza and Eidelberg, 1967), the volume of extracellular space was estimated to be 26.3%, which approaches the adult value of 21.7% (Fig. 2). These data agree closely with measurements of the maturing extracellular space based on uptake studies of tracers, water and electrolyte determinations and impedence measurements. They appeared to represent accurately the changing distribution of extracellular water during the course of development of a rapidly maturing cerebral cortex (Bondareff and Pysh, 1968) (Table 1).

Although the histophysiological significance of a progressively decreasing extracellular space cannot be accessed accurately, it is tempting to relate it to the onset of electrical activity. It is probable that these spaces contain a relatively large proportion of the extracellular water and chloride ion characteristic of the immature rat brain and that these extracellular channels facilitate diffusion of ions and metabolites. Such rapid diffusion of ions and small molecules through extracellular channels has been demonstrated in leech and amphibian nervous systems (Nicholls and Kuffler, 1964; Kuffler et al., 1966).

It is also probable that the extracellular channels contain macromolecules which facilitate, and perhaps control, the passage of ions and small molecules through them. That this extracellular substance is polyanionic has been suggested by several histochemical studies in which charged metallic complexes are visualized by electron microscopy, within the extracellular spaces. Such metallic substances include: ruthenium red (Bondareff, 1967a) (Fig. 3), phosphotungstic acid (Bloom and Aghajanian, 1966; Pease, 1966), bismuth iodide (Pfenninger *et al*., 1968), silver methenamine (Rambourg and Leblond, 1967) and uranyl acetate (Bondareff, 1967b). Because these substances are all positively charged, it has been assumed that their accumulation in tissues depends upon electrostatic forces binding them to anionic sites. The nature of these extracellular sites is not known precisely but it has been postulated that they may contain protein-bound mucopolysaccharide (acidic glycosaminoglycans) or glycoproteins (Pease, 1966; Bondareff, 1967 a, b; Bondareff and Sjöstrand, 1969). The possibility that these negatively charged macromolecules, which can bind water and selective ions reversibly, may influence neuronal excitability by affecting ionic fluxes at neuronal surfaces has been discussed before (Wang *et al*., 1966; Adey *et al*., 1969).

There is an apparent resemblance between brain extracellular space and the ground substance of connective tissues. Both appear to contain certain anionic substances that may be glycoproteins or mucopolysaccharides (Bondareff and Narotzky, 1972). Both appear to play prominent roles in normal histophysiology. Both undergo severe changes in water content and distribution during early development, and it is tempting to speculate that both may be profoundly changed as a consequence of normal aging. Because the ground substance of connective tissues condenses, becomes less hydrated, and is replaced by collagen as animals age (Bondareff, 1957; Joseph, 1971), we have been impelled to ask if the extracellular space of brain also changes during senescence.

We compared the volume of brain occupied by extracellular space in eight 26-month-old rats and in three 3-month-old animals (Bondareff and Narotzky, 1972). They were killed by decapitation after which the calvaria and dural membranes were rapidly removed, and the brain was exposed. A thin slice of cerebral cortex, from the parieto-occipital region near the midline, was excised and frozen rapidly. The frozen tissue water was substituted with a 1% solution of osmium tetroxide in absolute acetone at -78° C for 3 days, and the tissues were embedded in

Araldite-502. Sections, 0.5 µm thick, were cut perpendicular to the pial surface and examined with a light microscope. By this means, areas of the molecular layer of the cerebral cortex were identified in which damage due to ice crystal formation appeared minimal. These selected areas of tissue were isolated, sectioned at 500 to 700 A with an ultramicrotome and examined in an electron microscope. Five electron micrographs were prepared from each selected tissue area and the relative volume of extracellular space was estimated stereometrically in each (Weibel *et al.*, 1966).

The extracellular space appeared as lakes of variable dimension, which were noticeably smaller in tissues from the senescent animals. The mean volume of cerebral cortex occupied by extracellular space was 9.6 percent (range; 4.3 to 15.0 percent) in animals 26 months old (Fig. 4). In 3-month-old animals, the mean volume of cerebral cortex occupied by extracellular space was 20.8 percent (range; 18.7 to 22.3 percent) (Fig. 5), which agrees closely with our previously reported findings of a 21.7 percent mean volume of extracellular space in the cerebral cortices of four young adult female Sprague-Dawley rats (250 g each), prepared similarly by freeze-substitution (Bondareff and Pysh, 1968). The mean volumes of extracellular space for 3-month-old and 26-month-old rats were compared with a Mann-Whitney U test and a significant difference was suggested by a result of $P < .001$. These data are summarized in Table 2.

Since the brain contains essentially no connective tissue and the extracellular space appears to perform a histophysiological role comparable to that performed by connective tissue ground substance in non-neural organs (Gersh and Catchpole, 1960), a decreased capacity to transport ions and small molecules can reasonably be anticipated in the brains of senescent animals in which the volume occupied by extracellular space is reduced to about half that characteristic of normal adults (Bondareff and Narotzky, 1972). We have attempted to examine this speculation by comparing the capacity of brain tissue in old and young animals to transport exogenous catecholamines.

It had been shown that catecholamines, introduced into different specific brain loci in freely-moving rats through chronically-implanted cannulae, spread intracerebrally several millimeters from the point of application

(Bondareff et al., 1970). This can be demonstrated readily with catecholamines which can be visualized readily in brain tissue by the fluorescence histochemical method of Falck and Hillarp (Bondareff et al., 1970). We injected one group of female Sprague-Dawley rats intrastriatally with 1.0 µl of a solution containing 5.0 µg/µl dopamine-HCl dissolved in 150 mM NaCl and stabilized with ascorbic acid. A second group of animals was injected intrastriatally with 0.5 µl of DL-norepinephrine-HCl, 1.0 µg/µl, similarly prepared in 150 mM NaCl. The injections were made through stainless steel cannulae which had been implanted by stereotaxic surgery, 7 days previously into the right caudate nucleus. The animals were decapitated 15 minutes after the onset of the injection and their brains rapidly removed and frozen-dried. After condensation with formaldehyde vapors, the distribution of the exogenous catecholamines was determined in serial sections of the brains by fluorescence microscopy (Falck and Hillarp, 1962; Falck and Owman, 1965). We found no significant difference in intrastriatal spread of norepinephrine in non-senescent animals (1, 3, and 9 months of age), in which the spread varied between 0.45 mm and 0.54 mm rostral, and between 0.36 mm and 0.54 mm caudal to the point of application (Table 3). Total mean spread (rostral + caudal) in 7 non-senescent animals was 0.93 mm (range; 0.81 - 1.08 mm) and the difference between 1-month-old rats and those 3 and 9 months of age was not significant ($F=1.43$; $df=1,5$; $p<0.05$). The total spread for two 26-month-old senescent animals, however, was 0.45 mm and 0.54 mm (mean total spread = 0.50 mm), or almost half that observed in non-senescent animals (Table 3). This difference in spread between senescent and non-senescent animals was significant ($F=32.21$; $df=1,7$; $p<0.01$). Similarly, the total mean intrastriatal spread of dopamine (Table 4) in three senescent 24-month-old animals was 1.26 mm (range; 1.17 - 1.35 mm) (Bondareff et al., 1971), or about one half of that found in 6-month-old animals (Bondareff et al., 1970).

It cannot be claimed unequivocally that the decrease in intrastriatal spread of exogenous catecholamines in senescent rats to almost half that which is characteristic of non-senescent animals is associated with change in composition or volume of the extracellular space. But several data do support our tacit assumption that intrastriatal spread represents, at least in large part, an extracellular phenomenon. In the first place, the rate of intrastriatal spread, 0.5 mm/min is faster than that which has been ascribed to intracellular transport mechanisms (Routtenberg *et al.*, 1968); secondly, our observations that intrastriatal spread depends directly upon concentration suggests diffusion through extracellular channels (Bondareff *et al.*, 1970); and thirdly, the demonstration of reduced spread following pretreatment with dexamethosone or infusion with 20% mannitol (Bondareff *et al.*, 1970) is congruous with this assumption. Both dexamethosone pretreatment and infusion with 20% mannitol have been shown to decrease the volume of the extracellular space and to alter the normal relationship between intracellular and extracellular compartments in the brain. Both decrease intrastriatal spread by about half, suggesting further that spread is through extracellular channels.

Significant age-related decrements in both the volume of tissue occupied by extracellular space and in the capacity of brain tissue to transport exogenous catecholamines suggest an equally significant age-related change in the composition of the extracellular space. Analogy with connective tissue in non-neural organs suggests that such a change might best be sought in the constituent acidic glycosaminoglycans of extracellular proteoglycans which appear to occupy these extracellular spaces.

In preliminary studies of brains from 21-day and 24-month-old Sprague-Dawley rats, we have compared the acidic glycosaminoglycans by qualitative and quantitative methods well known to be useful in the comparison of young and old connective tissues (Breen *et al.*, 1970a, 1970b, 1973). Brains were lyophilized and defatted with chloroform-methanol, and the acidic glycosaminoglycans were isolated by ethanol precipitation after pronase digestion. Acidic glycosaminoglycan polymers were separated and identified by zone electrophoresis on cellulose acetate (Fig. 6) and quantitative measurements of uronic acid (U.A.), Hexosamine (Hex), galactosamine (Gal), and sulfate ($-SO_3^-$) were made (Table 5). Only apparently minor differences were found in the uronic acid and hexosamine contents of young and senescent brains. Similarly, only seemingly minor differences in total uronic acid and total chondroitin sulfate content were found. Yet, it may be significant that galactosamine content remained unchanged resulting in an apparent slight fall in the galactosamine per total hexosamine mole ratio in the brains of senescent animals (Table 6).

A prominent age-related change was found in the sulfate concentration of acidic glycosaminoglycans of old rats which was about 1-1/2 times greater than that of normal young brain (Table 5). If it is assumed that all the sulfate is on the galactosamine of chondroitin sulfates, an assumption strongly supported by our electrophoretic data, then the $-SO_3^-$:galactosamine mole ratio is 0.54 in 21-day-old rat brain as compared with 0.84 in senescent brain (Table 6). The relatively high $-SO_3^-$: galactosamine mole ratio in acidic glycosaminoglycans of senescent brains may reflect age-related changes in sulfotransferase activity or changes in the availability of sulfate acceptors, both of which appear to decrease with age (Balasubramanian and Bachawat, 1964; George *et al.*, 1970). There appears to be an age-related decrease in sulfate turnover with a consequent increase in sulfated chondroitin sulfates in senescent brain extracellular space but whether such changes are related to age-related changes in the neuronal microenvironment is not known.

The extracellular compartment of brain is composed largely of intercellular channels, which contain polyanions presumed to be proteoglycans. The dynamic microenvironment which this extracellular compartment provides to nerve cells has a histophysiological significance that is not well understood. That it has been shown to change with chronological age suggests that its properties during normal development and senescence may resemble those of the connective tissue ground substance and that it may affect a functional decline in the aging nervous system.

REFERENCES

Adey, W.R., Bystrom, B.G., Costin, A., Kado, R.T. and Tarby, T.J. (1969). *Exp. Neurol.* *23*, 29.

Balasubramanian, A.D. and Bachawat, B.K. (1964). *J. Neurochem.* *11*, 877.

Bloom, F.E. and Aghajanian, G.K. (1966). *Science* *154*, 1575.

Bondareff, W. (1957). *Gerontologia* *1*, 222.

Bondareff, W. (1967a). *Anat. Rec.* *157*, 527.

Bondareff, W. (1967b). *Z. Zellforsch.* *81*, 366.

Bondareff, W. and Narotzky, R. (1972). *Science* *176*, 1135.

Bondareff, W. and Pysh, J.J. (1968). *Anat. Rec.* *160*, 773.

Bondareff, W. and Sjöstrand, J. (1969). Exp. Neurol. 24, 450.
Bondareff, W. and Routtenberg, A., Narotzky, R. and McLone, D.G. (1970). Exp. Neurol. 28, 213.
Bondareff, W., Narotzky, R. and Routtenberg, A. (1971). J. Gerontol. 26, 163.
Breen, M., Weinstein, H.G., Andersen, M. and Veis, A. (1970a). Anal. Biochem. 35, 146.
Breen, M., Weinstein, H.G., Johnson, R.L., Veis, A. and Marshall, R.T. (1970b). Biochim. Biophys. Acta 201, 54.
Breen, M., Johnson, R.L., Sittig, R.A., Weinstein, H.G., Veis, A. and Marshall, R.T. (1973). Connective Tissue Res. (In press).
Bures, J. (1957). EEG Clin. Neurophysiol. 9, 121.
Deza, L. and Eidelberg, G. (1967). Exp. Neurol. 17, 425.
George, E., Singh, M. and Bachawat, B.K. (1970). J. Neurochem. 17, 189.
Gersh, I. and Catchpole, H.R. (1960). Perspectives Biol. Med. 3, 282.
Joseph. N.R. (1971). "Physical Chemistry of Ageing." Karger, Basel.
Horstmann, E. and Meves, H. (1959). Z. Zellforsch. 49, 569.
Koch, A. and Woodbury, D.M. (1960). Am. J. Physiol. 198, 434.
Kuffler, S.W., Nicholls, J.G. and Orkand, R.K. (1966). J. Physiol. 29, 768.
Malhotra, S.K. and Van Harreveld, A. (1966). J. Anat. 11, 99.
Margolis. R.U. (1967). Biochim. Biophys. Acta 141, 91.
Nicholls, J.G. and Kuffler, S.W. (1964). J. Physiol. 27, 645.
Pease, D.C. (1966). J. Ultrastruct. Res. 15, 555.
Pfenninger, K., Sandri, C., Akert, K. and Eugster, C.H. (1968). Brain Res. 12, 10.
Rambourg, A. and Leblond, C.P. (1967). J. Cell Biol. 32,27.
Reed, D.J. and Woodbury, D.M. (1960). Fed. Proc. 19, 80.
Routtenberg, A., Sladek, J. and Bondareff, W. (1968). Science 161, 272.
Schmitt, F.O. and Samson, F.E., Jr. (1969). Neurosci. Res. Program Bull. 7, 277.
Streicher, E. (1969). Am. J. Physiol. 201, 334.
Van Harreveld, A. (1966). Koninkl. Nederl. Akad. Van Weterschap. Series C 69, 17.
Van Harreveld, A., Collewijn, H. and Malhotra, S.K. (1966).

Am. J. Physiol. *210*, 251.

Van Harreveld, A., Crowell, J. and Malhotra, S.K. (1965). *J. Cell Biol.* *25*, 117.

Wang, H.H., Tarby, T.J., Kado, R.T. and Adey, W.R. (1966). *Science* *154*, 1183.

Weibel, E.R., Kistler, G.S. and Scherle, W.F. (1966). *J. Cell Biol.* *30*, 23.

Woodbury, D.M. (1958). *In* "Biology of Neuroglia" (W. F. Windle, ed.), pp. 120-127, Charles C. Thomas, Springfield, Illinois.

TABLE 1

Volume of extracellular space estimated in electron micrographs of frozen-substituted cerebral cortex of rats during early post-natal development.

Age	Number of animals	Extracellular space in %	
		Range	Mean
10 days	3	35.0-48.0	40.5
14 days	1	27.9-35.6	31.8
21 days	3	22.6-31.0	26.3
Adult	3	17.8-26.8	21.7

(From Bondareff and Pysh, 1968.)

TABLE 2

Estimated volume of extracellular space in electron micrographs of frozen-substituted cerebral cortex of rats, 26 and 3 months of age. Each estimate is based on the percentage of tissue volume occupied by extracellular space as estimated in five different electron microscopic fields. The average volumes are expressed as means ± standard deviation.

Rat (No.)	Volume per rat (%)
26 months old	
1	13.1±2.2
2	4.3±0.0
3	15.0±2.0
4	11.1±2.2
5	6.5±0.1
6	6.9±0.4
7	11.0±0.9
8	9.3±0.9
Average volume (%) per age group: 9.6±3.4	
3 months old	
9	18.7±1.5
10	22.3±1.7
11	20.6±1.1
Average volume (%) per age group: 20.8±1.5	

(Modified from Bondareff and Narotzky, 1972.)

TABLE 3

Relationship between chronological age and intrastriatal spread of 0.5 μl norepinephrine (1.0 μg/μl).

Rat #	Age (Mo.)	Spread (mm)		
		Rostral	Caudal	Total
5	1	0.54	0.36	0.90
6	1	0.45	0.54	0.99
7	1	0.54	0.54	1.08
1	1	0.45	0.54	0.99
9	3	0.45	0.36	0.81
4	3	0.45	0.36	0.81
12	9	0.54	0.45	0.99
10	9	0.18	0.27	0.45
11	26	0.27	0.27	0.54

(From Bondareff _et al._, 1970.)

TABLE 4

Relationship between chronological age and intrastriatal spread of 1.0 μl dopamine (5.0 μg/μl).

Rat #	Age (Mo.)	Spread (mm)		
		Rostral	Caudal	Total
20	6	1.08	1.22	2.30
35	6	0.72	2.07	2.79
55	6	0.45	0.72	1.17
74	24	0.54	0.81	1.35
75	24	0.54	0.72	1.26

(From Bondareff _et al._, 1970.)

TABLE 5

Acidic glycosaminoglycan polymers in whole brain of young and senescent rats.

Age (Mo.)	U.A.	Hex	Gal	$-SO_3^-$
	(μmole/g lipid-free dry weight)			
3	4.48	4.75	3.42	1.85
26	4.17	5.37	3.42	2.86

TABLE 6

Mole ratios of acidic glycosaminoglycan subunits from whole brain of young and senescent rats.

Age(Mo.)	U.A./HexN	GalN/HexN	$-SO_3^-$/HexN	$-SO_3^-$/GalN
3	0.94	0.72	0.39	0.54
26	0.78	0.64	0.53	0.84

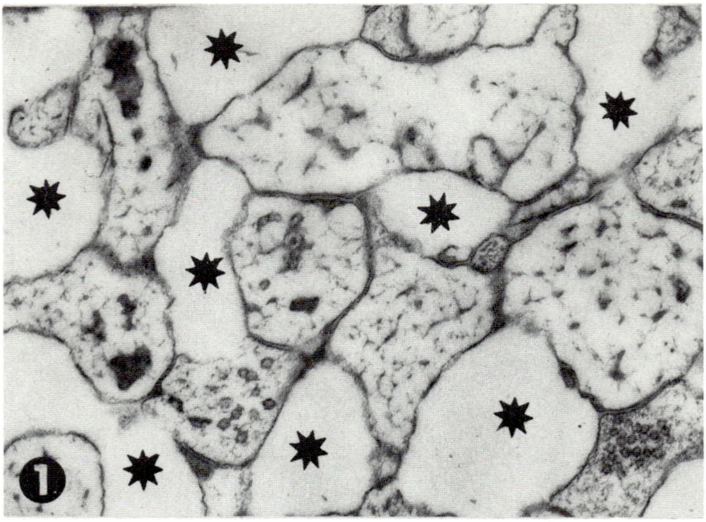

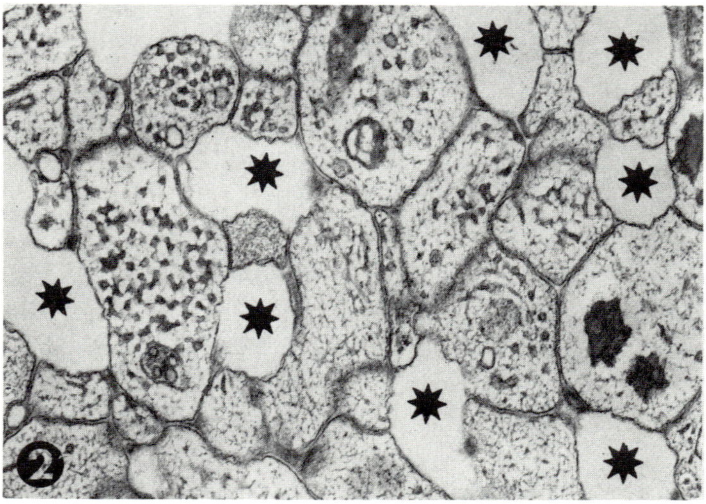

Figs. 1 and 2 Electron micrographs of frozen-substituted rat cerebral cortical neuropil demonstrating the relative distribution of the extracellular tissue compartment (indicated by stars). X35,000 (Modified from Bondareff and Pysh, 1968.)

Fig. 1 From an immature female, 10 days old. The volume of tissue occupied by extracellular space was estimated to be approximately 40%.

Fig. 2 From a young adult female, 3 months old. The volume of tissue occupied by extracellular space was estimated to be approximately 21%.

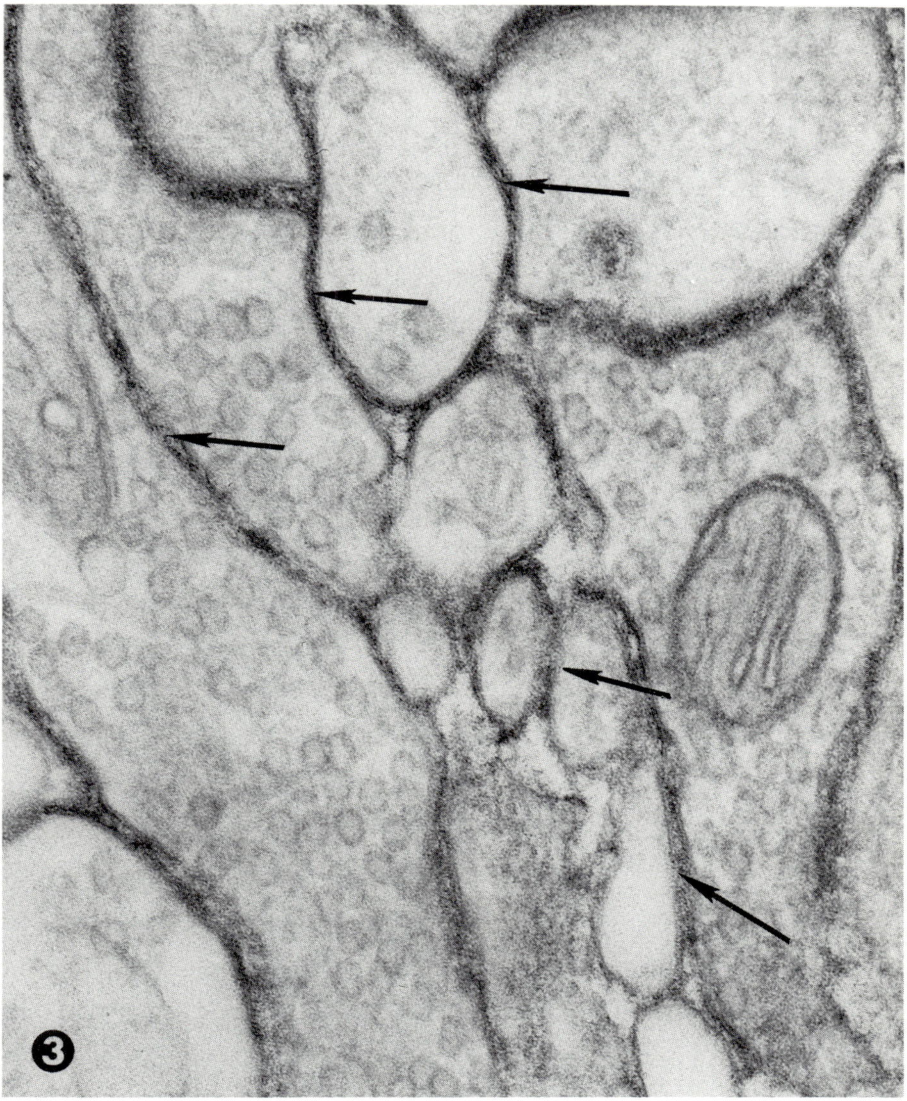

Fig. 3 Electron micrograph of rat cerebral cortical neuropil demonstrating ruthenium red reaction product in the extracellular tissue compartment (arrows). X122,400 (From Bondareff, 1967a.)

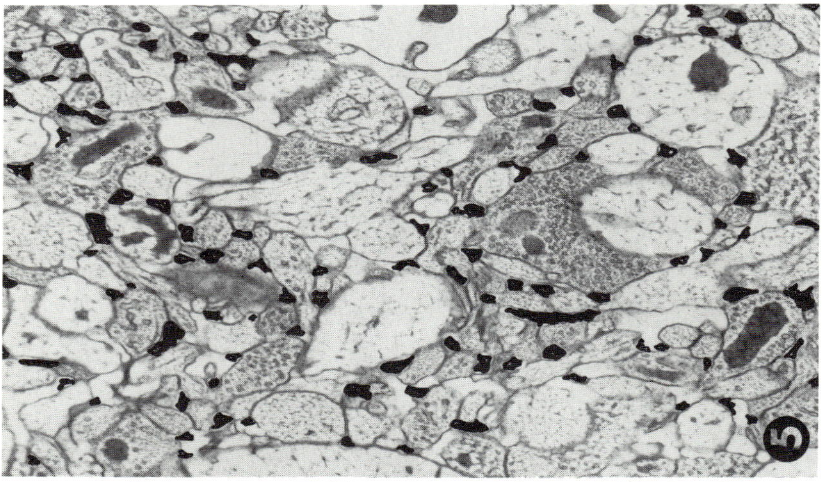

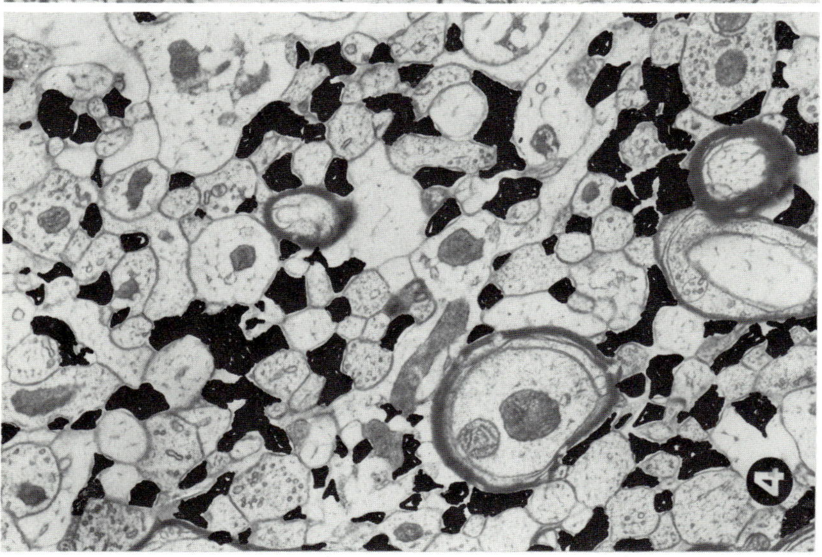

Fig. 4 and 5 caption on opposite page

Figs. 4 and 5 Electron micrographs of rat cerebral cortex fixed by freeze-substitution. The extracellular tissue compartment has been inked in. X18,000 (From Bondareff and Narotzky, 1972.)

Fig. 4 From a senescent female, 26 months old. The volume of tissue occupied by the extracellular space was estimated to be approximately 10%.

Fig. 5 From a young adult female, 3 months old. The volume of tissue occupied by extracellular space was estimated to be approximately 21%.

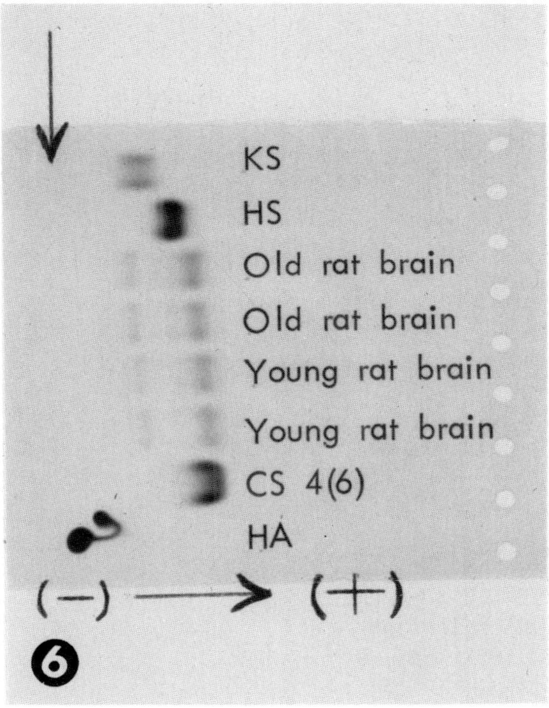

Fig. 6 Zone electrophoresis of acidic glycosaminoglycans isolated from whole rat brain and run in a phosphate buffer at pH 7.2. Vertical arrow indicates origin; horizontal arrow indicates direction of mobility. KS= keratan sulfate; HS=heparin sulfate; CS 4(6)=chondroitin sulfate 4(6); HA-hyaluronic acid.

NEURONAL DEATH AS A REGULATIVE MECHANISM IN THE CONTROL OF CELL NUMBER IN THE NERVOUS SYSTEM[1]

W. Maxwell Cowan

Department of Anatomy
Washington University School of Medicine
St. Louis, Missouri 63110

Among the many remarkable features of the nervous system, not the least is the apparent constancy in cell number of most fully developed neural systems. In certain invertebrate ganglia, where the numbers of neurons are quite small, this constancy is such that individual cells of known functional properties can be readily identified from animal to animal, even in the living state (for example, Nicholls and Baylor, 1969). In the vertebrate nervous system the very large numbers of cells make precise estimates of specific neuronal populations more difficult, but in those neural systems for which data are available, it appears that the numbers of neurons are remarkably constant. Several examples of this could be cited (Konigsmark, 1970), but two drawn from personal experience will serve to make the point. In the lateral mammillary nucleus of adult cats, the number of neurons on the two sides varies by no more than 9.3% and the average difference is on the order of 5% (Fry and Cowan, 1972). In the mesencephalic nucleus of the trigeminal nerve of the chick, which is small enough to permit accurate counts of the entire population, we have found that after the 13th day of incubation the number of cells on each side ranges from about 900 to 1,200, with a mean number of 1,035 (Rogers and Cowan, 1973).

While at first sight such constancy may seem not to

[1]Part of the work reported in this paper was supported by Grant 5 R01 EY 00599 from the National Institutes of Health.

be particularly surprising, it, in fact, suggests that there are rather precise control mechanisms acting to regulate cell number either during neurogenesis or in the period of neuronal maturation. At present these controls are quite obscure, but by analogy with what is known of the control of animal populations in the wild, we may be fairly certain that they involve a variety of interacting factors ranging from those which are genetic in the strictest sense to those which, in the broadest sense, may be termed morphogenetic. In this paper I propose to deal with only one of the latter, namely the role of neuronal death during normal development.

That cell death plays an important part in the development of other organs and tissues has been recognized for many years, and the evidence for it has been admirably reviewed by Glücksmann (1951). According to Glücksmann, such "normally occurring" cell degenerations may be considered histogenetic if their occurrence is an essential feature in the formation of a specific tissue, morphogenetic if they are responsible for shaping the final form of an organ or part, and phylogenetic if they represent, as it were, a recapitulation during ontogeny of an earlier phylogenetic sequence. While we may today question the validity of Glücksmann's third category, there can be little doubt that the first and second are of considerable significance throughout embryonic development, as Saunders, *et al.* (1962), Saunders (1966) and Saunders and Fallon (1966) have so convincingly shown. Considerations of space forbid a thorough discussion of these more general aspects of the problem, but they are mentioned here since it has become evident that the widespread (and possibly universal) occurrence of neuronal death during the normal development of the central and peripheral nervous system is but one example of what now appears to be a general developmental principle.

That cell death may be one of the major factors determining neuronal number, and in this way of neural organization as a whole, has only recently been appreciated. Yet the earliest observations of degenerating cells in the developing nervous system were reported more than 60 years ago (Collin, 1906); moreover, scattered throughout the literature of the past half century there are many isolated references to the appearance of degenerating neurons in the brains of various embryos or to a progressive decline in neuronal number in certain neural systems during the course of ontogeny. However, it is only in the past decade or so that the magnitude of this phenomenon and its widespread occurrence in the brains of most classes of vertebrates, and in many different neural systems, have been recognized, largely as a result of the work of Hughes (1961, 1965) and Prestige (1965, 1967), who have devoted a good deal of attention to this issue in the developing amphibian spinal cord and spinal ganglia.

Since their work has been reviewed *in extenso* in two recent monographs (Hughes, 1968; Prestige, 1970), it will suffice here to say that they have found that there is normally a considerable over-production of neurons in the motor columns of the cord and in the spinal ganglia, as judged by the fact that the number of neurons present in both regions at early larval stages is appreciably greater than the number recognizable after metamorphosis. Serial counts of the number of cells indicate that there is a marked loss in both the motor columns and the spinal ganglia coincident with the onset of limb movements, and during this critical period (between stages 54 and 59 in *Xenopus*) large numbers of degenerating cells can be seen in both regions. By estimating the additional number of degenerating cells seen after limb ablations, Hughes has calculated that the rate of neuronal death in the spinal cord may be of the order of 3.2 hours, and that if the "normally occurring" cell degeneration occurs at the same rate, at least eight neurons must degenerate for every one that survives to maturity. This implies that during the larval period there must be an appreciable "turnover" of cells in the amphibian nervous system such that new neurons are continually being added to the population while others are degenerating.

While one may question Hughes' conclusions regarding the magnitude of this turnover (since it is not immediately apparent that the rate of neuronal degeneration during normal development should be the same as that after limb removal) there can be little doubt that cell death is a major factor determining neuron number in the anuran nervous system. However, since there appear to be a number of important differences in the pattern of neurogenesis between amphibians and amniotes, it is not clear whether we can generalize from these observations of cell loss in the amphibian spinal cord and ganglia, and the question remains whether cell death plays a significant morphogenetic role in the nervous system of higher vertebrates.

As yet, too little is known about the development of the mammalian nervous system from this point of view, to answer such questions definitively. There are a few scattered reports in the literature which suggest that at least some degree of cell loss is a normal concomitant of neural development in mammals. For example, Romanes (1946) has reported a progressive loss of cells from the motor columns of the ventral horn of normal mice amounting to about 30% between the 2nd and the 12th days postnatally. More recently, Harris (1965) has shown that the formation of discrete ventral horns at the non-limb levels of the mouse spinal cord is due to the morphogenetic death of a substantial number of neurons. It is probable that further study of the developing mammalian nervous system will bring to light several more examples of this phenomenon, but because of the difficulties inherent in the experimental manipulation of mammalian fetuses (Hess, 1957) it is unlikely that a critical analysis of the significance of cell death in controlling neuronal number in the mammalian central nervous system will be forthcoming for some time.

By contrast, there is already a very substantial body of evidence to suggest that during the development of the avian nervous system, cell death occurs rather widely and that it plays a critical morphogenetic role in shaping many neural centers. The first clear demonstration of this was presented in the seminal study of Hamburger and Levi-Montalcini (1949) who showed that during normal development there is a very substantial neuronal degeneration in the dorsal root ganglia of the chick at cervical and thoracic levels and that most of the difference in the size of these ganglia and those at the brachial and lumbo-sacral levels is directly attributable to this morphogenetic cell loss. Not only is this degeneration topographically patterned in that it affects certain ganglia while apparently sparing others, it also follows a distinctive temporal sequence. The earliest degenerations are found in the most rostral ganglia (at about 4-1/2 days) and it is not until the 6th day that a significant number of degenerating cells are found at the lower sacral levels. Moreover, it seems to affect principally the large ventrolaterally located ganglion cells (which are the first neurons to be differentiated in the ganglia) and, by and large, does not involve the smaller dorsomedially placed cells. The similarity in the topographic distribution of this "normally occurring" neuronal degeneration and that seen after extirpation of the limb buds led them to suggest that the same underlying mechanism was responsible, namely, a limitation in the extent of the available peripheral innervation field. Or, to express it differently, the survival of so many large ventrolateral ganglion cells at the brachial and lumbo-sacral segments during normal development is directly attributable to the presence of the fore- and hind-limbs and the expanded peripheral innervation fields which they represent. The fact that more of these cells survive after the transplantation of a supernumerary limb, may be regarded as further evidence in support of this view.

An even more striking example of morphogenetic cell death was presented by Levi-Montalcini (1950) in her study of the development of the visceral (i.e., the preganglionic sympathetic) system in the chick. Until about the end of the 3rd day of incubation there are no significant regional differences in the motor columns of the spinal cord. However, during the 4th day there is an impressive secondary migration of cells from the ventral motor columns (especially at thoracic and lumbar levels) which, in time, leads to the formation of a distinct viscero-motor nucleus. Concurrent with the onset of this neuronal migration there is a large scale degeneration of neurons in the ventral horn at cervical levels. Although this phase of degeneration only lasts for about 12 hours, it results in the complete disappearance of the abortive visceral system in the cervical region. At its peak, the degeneration is said to be so severe as to temporally obscure the presence of the intact cells.

In a later study of the development of the motor columns of the cord and the effects of early limb bud ablation, Hamburger (1958) showed rather clearly that, even in the brachial and lumbo-sacral segments, some neuronal degeneration normally takes place and, in the case of the brachial segments, this "normally occurring" degeneration reaches its peak at about the same time as the much more dramatic cell breakdown that occurs after removal of the wing bud. While the identification of degenerating cells at the light microscope level is not always easy (and where the number of degenerating cells is small, some doubt may exist as to their significance), with the electron microscope the appearance of the degenerating cells is quite unequivocal (Bodian, 1966). Figure 1, which is taken from an unpublished study of the development of the cervical cord in the chick by Dr. Robert Skoff, shows rather clearly the progressive nuclear pycnosis which is so characteristic of degeneration in immature neurons and the subsequent phagocytosis of the neuronal debris by the surrounding glial cells.

My own attention was first drawn to the importance of cell death during neural development in 1965 when, in association with Dr. Eleanor Wenger, I began a series of studies on the development of the avian visual system and the effects of early eye removal. Since our optic vesicle and optic cup extirpations included varying amounts of the extraocular mesoderm from which the extrinsic eye muscles were formed, we were interested in examining the changes in the eye motor nuclei of the brainstem. The trochlear nucleus was of particular interest because its small size and clear cytoarchitectonic differentiation permitted us to estimate fairly accurately the number of cells in the nucleus at several developmental stages. To our surprise, we found that not only was there a progressive loss of neurons from the nucleus on the side contralateral to the eye removal, but towards the end of the incubation period the control nucleus also showed a significant reduction in cell number. Figure 2, which is taken from that study (Cowan and Wenger, 1967), shows that at the 9th day of incubation the chick trochlear nucleus contains about 1,300 cells, but during the latter half of the incubation period this number declines steadily to a definitive population of between 500 and 650. Since most of the cells in the nucleus are generated, i.e., pass through their last phase of DNA synthesis on the 3rd day of incubation (Cowan, unpublished observations) and since, as Dunnebacke (1953) had earlier shown, the nucleus is numerically complete on the 5th day of incubation, it would appear that all the neurons in the nucleus are capable of surviving for at least 7 or 8 days. In the ensuing 10 or 12 days about 50-60% of the cells degenerate at the rate of about 60 per day. Probably because of their slow rate of fallout and the rapidity which the cells degenerated or were removed from the nucleus, there was little overt sign of cell degeneration in the trochlear nucleus. However, the consistency of the cell counts after the 17th day of incubation leaves no doubt as to the reality of this morphogenetic cell death. Again, the similarity in the time course of this normally occurring cell loss and the greatly accentuated cell loss which occurred after removal of some of the extraocular mesoderm, suggested that the extent of the available innervation field was the limiting factor determining the size of the definitive neuronal population.

A second example of cell death during the development of the visual system was found in our study of the nucleus of origin of centrifugal fibers to the retina (Cowan and Wenger, 1968). The cells in this nucleus - the so-called isthmo-optic nucleus - arise on the 6th or 7th days of incubation (Hart, 1969) and by day 11 they form a rather compact, ovoid mass of cells in the dorsolateral part of the caudal midbrain. At this stage the nucleus has no distinctive cytoarchitectonic appearance (Fig. 3) and has been found to contain approximately 27,000 cells. Over the course of the next few days, but especially between days 13 and 17, the compact mass of cells becomes converted into the highly convoluted sheet characteristic of the adult nucleus (Fig. 4) by a dramatic, and highly patterned, wave of neuronal degeneration. As the result of this, the number of cells in the nucleus is reduced by about 60%, to a definitive population of about 11,000 neurons. Since during the critical period between the 13th and 15th days of incubation cells in the nucleus are degenerating at a rate of 200-300 per hour, considerable numbers of cells with pycnotic nuclei and disintegrating perikarya can be seen in the central portion of the nucleus at this time. Following the earlier removal of the contralateral optic vesicle or optic cup the "normally occurring" cell loss is greatly accentuated and leads within a very short time to the total disappearance of the nucleus.

Perhaps the most significant feature of the "normally occurring" cell death in the isthmo-optic nucleus is its highly ordered spatial pattern. Although this is not apparent during the period of maximum cell death or in the gross morphology of the mature nucleus, it is evident in the high degree of organization which exists in the projection of the nucleus upon the contralateral retina. McGill, *et al.* (1966a, b) have shown from reconstructions of the nucleus in adult pigeons that, despite its apparent folding, the nucleus can be considered as a continuous sheet of cells, so arranged as to provide a complete, and precisely arranged, retino-topic projection. This means that during its development from an amorphous neuronal mass to its mature form, a very specific pattern of cell degeneration must occur, and that this pattern must reflect very accurately the spatial distribution of the amacrine and displaced ganglion cells upon which the axons of the isthmo-optic cells terminate (Cowan, 1970; Holden and Powell, 1972). Just how this is brought about is difficult to envision, but that the development of the appropriate retinal neurons plays a decisive role in the selection of the surviving isthmo-optic cells is strongly suggested by the localized areas of complete cell loss which occur in the nucleus after partial ablations of the developing retina (see Cowan and Wenger, 1968, and Fig. 4). Unfortunately, until we know when the isthmo-optic fibers reach the retina and, more importantly, when they normally establish synaptic contact with their target neurons, definitive evidence on this issue will be lacking.

Although it seems somewhat implausible, a possible criticism of many of the studies, in which a pattern of neuronal degeneration has been inferred from successive cell counts, is that much of the apparent disappearance of neurons is due to the misidentification, at the earliest stages, of cells which later will become more clearly recognizable as neuroglia. One neural system in which this can be effectively ruled out is the mesencephalic nucleus of the trigeminal nerve. The reason for this is that within just a few days of their generation the cells of this nucleus take on their characteristic unipolar form; since they are among the largest nerve cells in the midbrain, their identification presents no problem. In the chick the cells of the mesencephalic nucleus arise from the region of the neural folds between the 3rd and 4th days of incubation, and by the 6th day most of the cells have migrated to their definite location, either in the tectal commissure or in one of the deeper layers of the optic tectum (Rogers and Cowan, 1973). At this time, the nucleus on each side contains a total of about 4,000-4,500 cells, arranged in two groups - medial and lateral - and the population seems stable until the 9th day of incubation. However, in the succeeding 4 days, and especially between days 11 and 13, there is a marked degeneration of cells in both parts of the nucleus, so that by the 13th day the number of cells is reduced to just over 1,000. From the 13th day of incubation onwards there is no significant change in the number of cells in the nucleus (at least until the 3rd week after hatching, see Fig. 5) but, of course, the individual neurons continue to grow for some time.

Because the cells of the mesencephalic nucleus are spread out over such a considerable mediolateral and rostrocaudal extent, the identification of degenerating neurons at any one stage is rather difficult; but during the period of maximum cell loss (between days 11 and 13) a number of identifyably degenerating neurons have definitely been seen, especially in the rostral part of the nucleus (Fig. 6).

The loss of almost 75% of the cells originally seen in the mesencephalic nucleus makes this one of the most striking examples of a normally occurring cell loss in the avian central nervous system. Moreover, it is interesting to note that the neuronal degeneration is not uniformly distributed throughout the nucleus. Serial plots of the numbers of cells in successive sections through the rostro-caudal extent of the nucleus in embryos before the 10th day of incubation show two distinct peaks in the neuron population; one in its rostral third and a second at its caudal end (Fig. 7). After the period of cell loss the rostral peak is markedly reduced, but the caudal peak is completely eliminated. The significance of this selective loss of cells from the caudal part of the nucleus is not known at present and will be difficult to determine until the peripheral distribution of the fibers of the mesencephalic root of V has been established. Nevertheless, the consistency of this pattern of cell loss from animal to animal seems to signify that, as in the dorsal root ganglia and the motor columns of the spinal cord, the process of cell degeneration is spatially programmed in a rather precise manner.

The sequence of innervation of the jaw musculature in the chick does not appear to have been studied. If it should turn out that the development of muscle spindles in the head region is comparable to that in the limbs, there would be an interesting temporal coincidence between the time of occurrence of the cell loss in the mesencephalic nucleus and the period of spindle formation. According to Tello (1922) muscle spindle formation in the limbs begins on the 9th day of incubation; by the 11th and 12th days individual spindles are clearly recognizable, and no new spindles are formed after the 13th day. If it could be shown that a similar sequence occurs during the innervation of the jaw muscles, we should have strong reasons for thinking that the cell loss in the mesencephalic nucleus is due to a limitation in the number of available spindles in its innervation field, such that the majority of the cells are unable to form appropriate peripheral connections. Support for this view may be found in the experiments of Piatt (1946) in _Ambystoma_, and of Rogers and Cowan (1973) in the chick, in which large portions of the presumptive jaw mesoderm were ablated. In both studies this operation resulted in a marked reduction in the final number of cells in the mesencephalic nucleus of V, amounting in some cases to as much as 60 to 70%. But of even greater interest is Piatt's (1946) finding that the transplantation of additional jaw mesoderm in _Ambystoma_ larvae may lead to a substantial _hyperplasia_ in the mesencephalic nucleus. At present it is not known if this is attributable to a stimulatory effect on cell proliferation or to the regulation of cell death, and regrettably it has not been possible, to date, to repeat these experiments in the chick. If it could be shown that an enlargement of the innervation field of the mesencephalic nucleus (possibly by the heteroplastic transplantation of the large mandibular lobe of ducks into chick embryos) results in the survival of an appreciably larger number of neurons in the nucleus, this would perhaps provide the strongest evidence that the periphery normally plays an important role in regulating cell survival in the nervous system.

A number of other examples of cell death during normal development could be given, were space available, but enough has already been said to indicate that the phenomenon is both extremely widespread and of considerable significance in controlling the total number of neurons in most, if not all, neuronal populations and also in molding the final form of certain neural centers. It is difficult at this time to do more than document the observation that the phenomenon is a real one; much further work will be needed before we can answer most of the critical questions which these descriptive studies have raised.

Among the questions to which we should like answers are:

1) Is this a general phenomenon in the sense that it is common to all nervous systems, vertebrate and invertebrate, and affects all, or most, neural populations?

2) Even if it is not a universal phenomenon, why should there be such a gross overproduction of nerve cells in so many neural centers, and is the cell death that occurs truly "programmed" or is it largely fortuitous?

3) Are most peripheral effects on early neural development due to the regulation of neuronal death and, if so, to what extent can the size of a neuronal population be increased by reducing the level of cell loss?, and

4) Finally, what is the signal that triggers the death of so many cells, and how do other cells in the same population escape this influence?

Unfortunately, as in most areas of neurobiology, it is easy to pose such questions, but difficult to answer them, or even to suggest ways in which they may be answered. It may be helpful, nevertheless, to discuss these and other questions and, in doing so, to indicate the types of further evidence that are needed and certain hypotheses which are compatible with the available evidence.

1) As we have seen, in virtually every neural system whose development has been carefully analyzed from this point of view, there has been some indication of a "normally occurring" cell loss. I have purposely limited myself to a consideration of the vertebrate nervous system, but the same generalization may well be made for invertebrates (see Nordlander and Edwards, 1968). Although even among the vertebrates reliable information is largely limited to certain anurans and the chick, there seems no reason to doubt that similar observations will, in time, be made in other classes of vertebrates. It would be particularly interesting to know to what extent it occurs in nervous systems of mammals in general and in the human nervous system in particular. It should not be difficult to answer this for most of the common laboratory mammals by examining certain well-defined nuclear groups such as the cranial nerve nuclei, at successive periods in development. Now that human fetal material is becoming increasingly accessible, it may be possible, at least at the descriptive level, to obtain comparable evidence for the human nervous system.

2) It is difficult to know why nature should apparently be so profligate in the production of neurons. In some

of the systems I have discussed, as many as eight cells are generated for every one that survives to maturity, and even if we exclude those situations in which there may be a turnover of neurons, the initial number of cells produced often seems to exceed the final number by a factor of 2 or 3. Until we can effectively rule out that the cells which die do not serve some transient function in the economy of the developing nervous system, it may be misleading to speak of an "overproduction" of neurons, but from the evidence that we have at present this certainly seems to be the case. Certainly in most systems the cells which die and those which survive are indistinguishable on the basis of their perikaryal morphology up to the critical period when the first neuronal degeneration begins. Of course, an examination of the cells' perikarya tells us very little, and in trying to assess a possible transient function for the cells which fail to survive, it may be much more important to know something of the status of their axonal and dendritic processes. For example, in most of the situations I have described it is not known whether the fated cells send out axons to their projection fields and in most of them it is quite impossible to carry out the requisite, serial fiber counts. Fortunately this is not the case in the anuran spinal cord and Prestige and Wilson (1972) have recently addressed themselves to this important question. By counting the numbers of axons identifiable in electron micrographs of the ventral roots of _Xenopus_ at representative stages of development, they have been able to show that there is an approximately 1:1 correspondence between the numbers of such fibers and the numbers of motoneurons in the corresponding spinal segment. While it is impossible to rule out that some of the fibers counted in the ventral roots may be due to axonal branching, the fact that the total number of fibers in the 9th ventral root drops from about 2,000 at stage 54 to just over 500 at stage 55 and, thereafter, remains fairly constant through metamorphosis, suggests rather strongly that during axonal development most motoneurons send out axons to the periphery and that the causative factors responsible for the death of a substantial number of them is to be found, not within the motoneuron pool, but in the circumstances prevailing at the periphery.

There may well be several critical factors operating in the cells' peripheral innervation field, but of these the most significant seems to be the inability of the outgrowing axons to form the appropriate peripheral relationship, be it with a group of sensory receptors, muscle fibers, gland cells, or other neurons. There are two impelling reasons for this view: first there is the striking similarity in time of occurrence of the "normal" cell loss and the greatly accentuated neuronal degeneration that follows early ablation of the peripheral field; and, secondly, the "normally occurring" cell loss seems to take place in most systems at the time when we have reason to believe that peripheral connections are being established. Unfortunately, we know all too little about the precise timing of synaptogenesis or peripheral innervation, and almost nothing about the numbers of available postsynaptic cells or peripheral receptors during development. But if we are correct in thinking that a proportion of the cells in most neural populations degenerate because their axons are unable to find appropriate peripheral "targets", it would seem that there must be some sort of competition between the outgrowing axons for the available contact sites, comparable to that which has recently been postulated for the feline visual system (Guillery, 1972) and the rat dentate gyrus (Gottlieb and Cowan, 1972). That is to say, the final determination of cell number in the nervous system may be a matter of "the survival of the fittest" - where the fitness of the neurons is defined as their ability to establish contacts which are appropriate, both in type and number. Whatever "programming" is involved in the establishment of neural connections must relate to the population as a whole rather than to individual neurons within the population.[2]

3) Neuroembryologists have, for some time, been divided on the issue of whether or not the periphery can regulate cell proliferation in the developing nervous system. Since I have dealt with this problem in some detail elsewhere (Kelly and Cowan, 1972) and have alluded to it above, it will suffice here to say that there is little evidence to support the view that the periphery can influence the proliferation of neurons (as opposed to glia) and in some systems such an influence can be definitely ruled

[2]It is, of course, impossible to rule out that certain neurons within the population are "mis-specified" and hence incapable of forming appropriate connections.

out (De Long and Sidman, 1962; Scalia and Cowan, 1973). This means that the only way in which the periphery can effectively control neural development in these systems is by the regulation of cell survival. Since, in many neural systems, neuronal proliferation ceases long before the cells are in a position to establish peripheral connections the "overproduction" of neurons within a center clearly confers a considerable advantage upon that center, enabling it to accommodate, as it were, a fairly wide range of variation within its innervation field. We have known for a long time that a reduction in the size of a peripheral field permits fewer neurons to survive; what we really need is a careful study of peripheral overloading to establish unequivocally that the enlargement of a peripheral field promotes the survival of a larger-than-normal neuronal population.

4) By analogy with the neuronal degeneration that occurs in a neuronal center after ablating a portion of its peripheral innervation field, the normally occurring cell loss is commonly thought of as a form of retrograde degeneration. The notion behind this is that the failure of the axons to establish an appropriate connection is in some way 'signalled' back to the neuronal somata. But just what the nature of this signal is, and how a neuron senses that its axon has, or has not, established a connection is quite unknown. It has been postulated that there is an actual transfer of material from the target cell or tissue to the axon and that the materials taken up by the axon terminals are conveyed back to the neuronal soma by a retrograde axoplasmic transport. Obviously, if the survival of a neuron is dependent upon a constant supply of such trophic substances, any neuron which was unsuccessful in establishing a trophic relationship with the appropriate target cells would, in time, degenerate. But, like the similar suggestion that it is the continual supply of materials <u>from</u> an axon <u>to</u> the cells with which it is in contact that is essential for maintenance of the parent neuron, this hypothesis is purely speculative and, at present, has no substantive basis.

REFERENCES

Bodian, D. (1966). *Bull. Johns Hopkins Hosp.* **119**, 212.
Collin, R. (1906). *Le Nevraxe* **8**, 185.

Cowan, W.M. and Wenger, E. (1967). J. Exp. Zool. 164, 267.
Cowan, W.M. and Wenger, E. (1968). J. Comp. Neurol. 133, 207.
Cowan, W.M. (1970). Brit. Med. Bull. 26, 112.
De Long, G.R. and Sidman, R.L. (1962). J. Comp. Neurol. 118,205.
Dunnebacke, T.H. (1953). J. Comp. Neurol. 98, 155.
Fry, F.J. and Cowan, W.M. (1972). J. Comp. Neurol. 144, 1.
Glücksmann, A. (1951). Biol. Rev. 26, 59.
Gottlieb, D.I. and Cowan, W.M. (1972). Brain Res. 41, 452.
Guillery, R.W. (1972). J. Comp. Neurol. 144, 117.
Hamburger, V. and Levi-Montalcini, R. (1949). J. Exp. Zool. 111, 457.
Hamburger, V. (1958). Amer. J. Anat. 102, 365.
Harris, A.E. (1965). Cited in Prestige (1970).
Hart, J. (1969). "Some observations on the development of the avian optic tectum." Ph.D. Thesis, University of Wisconsin.
Hess, A. (1957). Biol. Rev. 32, 231.
Holden, A.L. and Powell, T.P.S. (1972). J. Physiol.(Lond.) 223, 419.
Hughes, A. (1961). J. Embryol. exp. Morphol. 9, 269.
Hughes, A. (1965). J. Embryol. exp. Morphol. 13, 9.
Hughes, A. (1968). "Aspects of Neural Ontogeny." Academic Press, New York.
Kelly, J.P. and Cowan, W.M. (1972). Brain Res. 42, 263.
Konigsmark, B.W. (1970). In "Contempory Research Methods in Neuroanatomy" (W.J.H. Nauta and S.O.E. Ebbesson, eds.), pp. 315-339, Springer-Verlag, New York.
Levi-Montalcini, R. (1950). J. Morphol. 86, 253.
McGill, J.I., Powell, T.P.S. and Cowan, W.M. (1966a). J. Anat. (Lond.) 100, 5.
McGill, J.I., Powell, T.P.S. and Cowan, W.M. (1966b). J. Anat. (Lond.) 100, 35.
Nicholls, T. and Baylor, D.A. (1969). Endeavour 28, 3.
Nordlander, R.H. and Edwards, J.S. (1968). Nature 218,780.
Piatt, J. (1946). J. Exp. Zool. 102, 109.
Prestige, M.C. (1965). J. Embryol. exp. Morphol. 13, 63.
Prestige, M.C. (1967). J. Embryol. exp. Morphol. 18, 359.
Prestige, M.C. (1970). In "The Neurosciences" (F.O.Schmitt, ed.), pp. 73-82, Rockefeller Univ. Press, New York.
Prestige, M.C. and Wilson, M.A. (1972). Brain Res. 41, 467.
Rogers, L.A. and Cowan, W.M. (1973). J. Comp. Neurol. 147, 291.

Romanes, G.J. (1946). J. Anat, (Lond.) 80, 117.
Saunders, J.W. (1966). Science 154, 604.
Saunders, J.W. and Fallon, J.F. (1966). In "Major Problems in Development Biology" (M. Locke, ed.), pp. 289-314, Academic Press, New York.
Saunders, J.W., Gasseling, M.T. and Saunders, L.C. (1962). Develop. Biol. 5, 147.
Scalia, J.C. and Cowan, W.M. (1973). In preparation.
Skoff, R. (1973). Personal communication.
Tello, J.T. (1922). Z. ges. Anat. u. Z. Anat. Entw. Gesch. 64, 348.

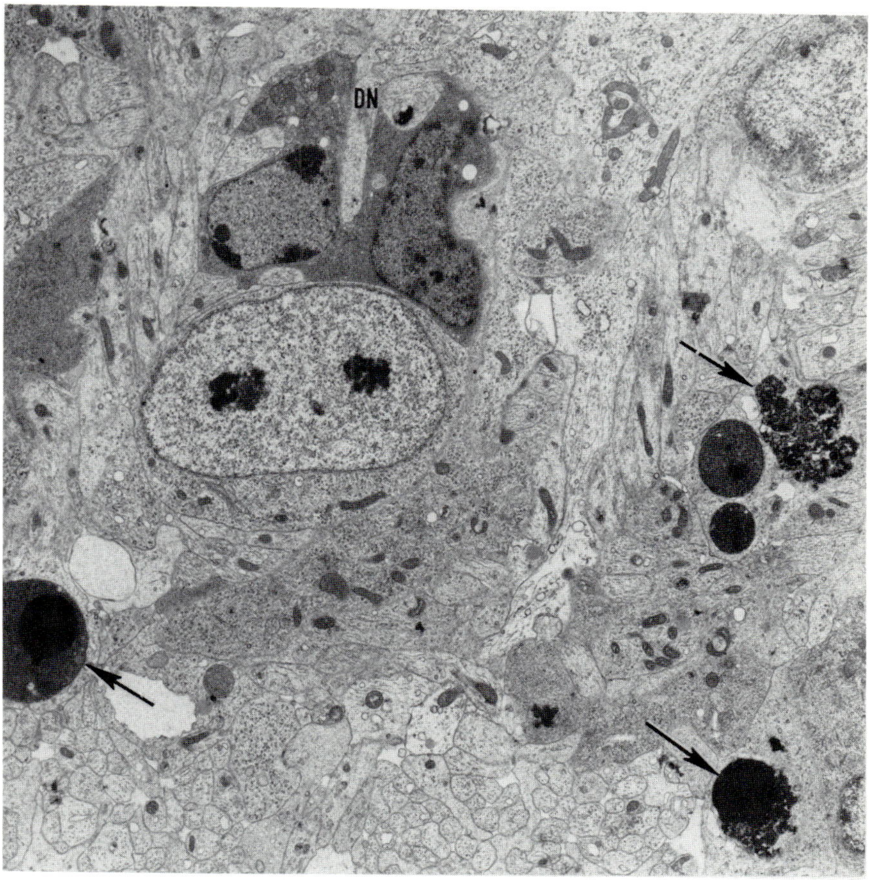

Fig. 1 An electron micrograph of the cervical cord of a normal 4-1/2 day chick embryo, prepared by Dr. Robert Skoff, to show the appearance of neurons in various stages of degeneration, from those showing only minimal nuclear pycnosis (DN) to the final ingestion of the neuronal debris by glial cells (arrows) X15,120

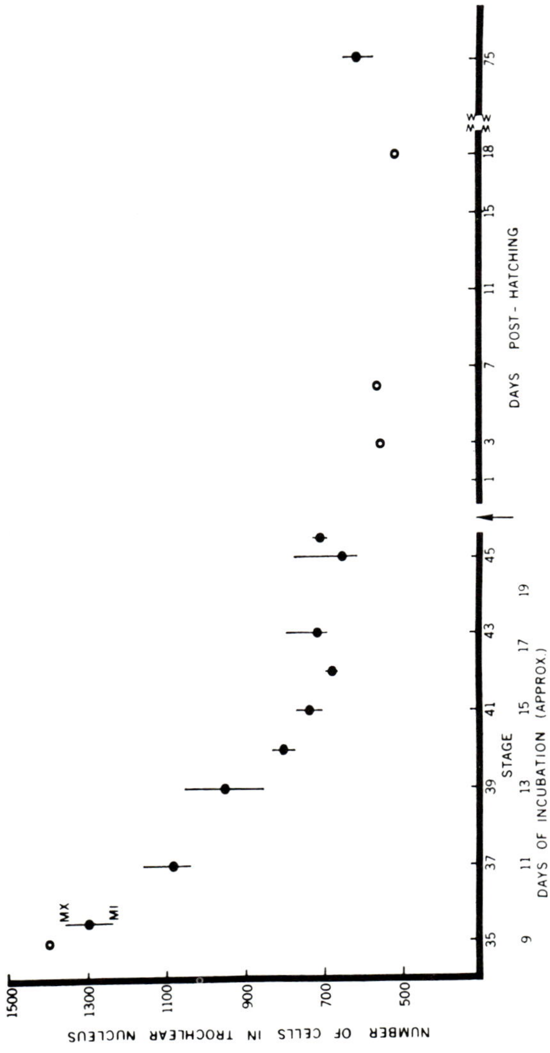

Fig. 2 The progressive loss of neurons during the normal development of the trochlear nucleus of the chick is shown. (From Cowan and Wenger, 1967.)

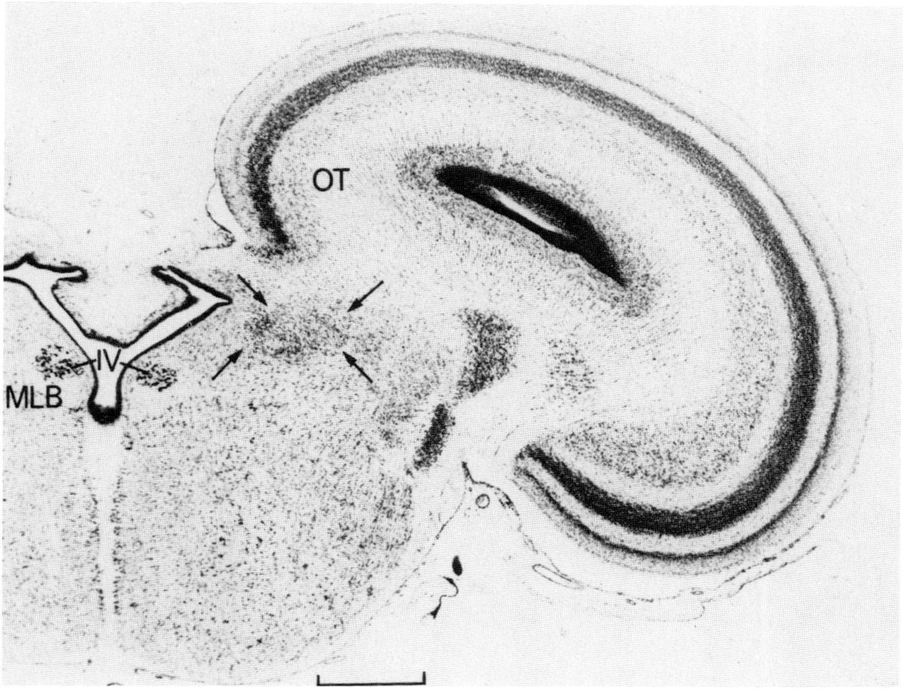

Fig. 3 The appearance of the isthmo-optic nucleus of the chick at the 11th day of incubation. At this stage the nucleus contains about 27,000 cells compactly arranged and with little or no evidence of cytoarchitectonic organization. MLB: medial longitudinal bundle; IV: trochlear nucleus; OT: optic tectum. Scale: 0.5 mm. (From Cowan and Wenger, 1968.)

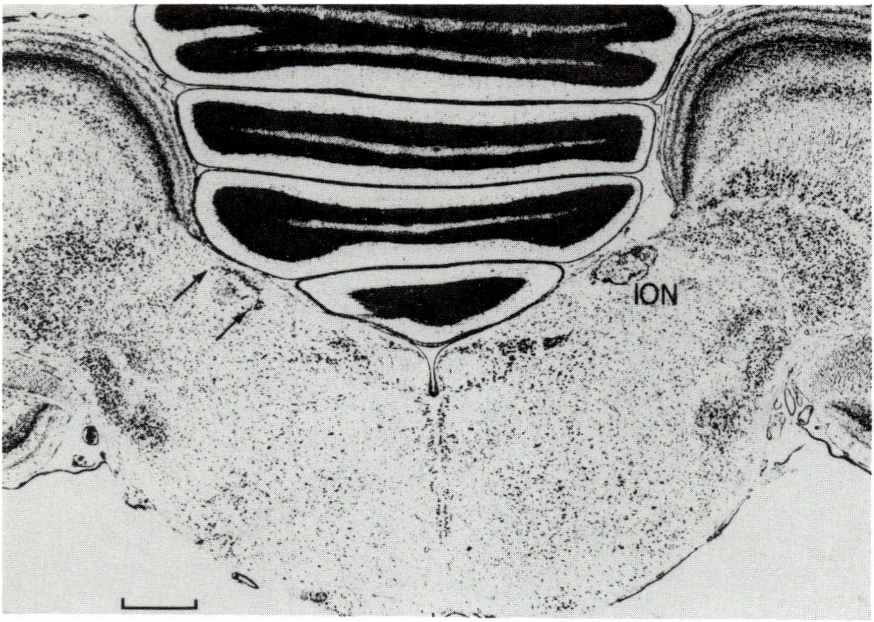

Fig. 4 On the right is the normal isthmo-optic nucleus (ION) as it appears in a mature chick; at this stage the nucleus contains only about 11,000 cells (cf. Fig. 3). The nucleus on the left side of the photomicrograph shows a clear zone of cell loss (marked by the arrows) in its ventral portion. This was due to the removal early in the 3rd day of incubation of a large part of the developing optic cup. Scale: 0.5 mm. (From Cowan and Wenger, 1968.)

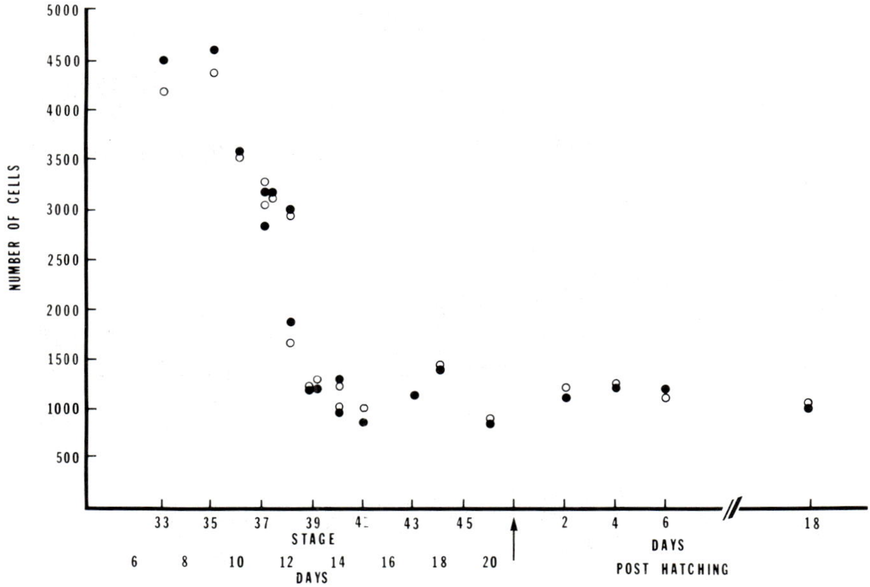

Fig. 5 A graph to show the dramatic cell loss which normally occurs in the mesencephalic nucleus of the trigeminal nerve of the chick between the 9th and 13th days of incubation. (From Rogers and Cowan, 1973.)

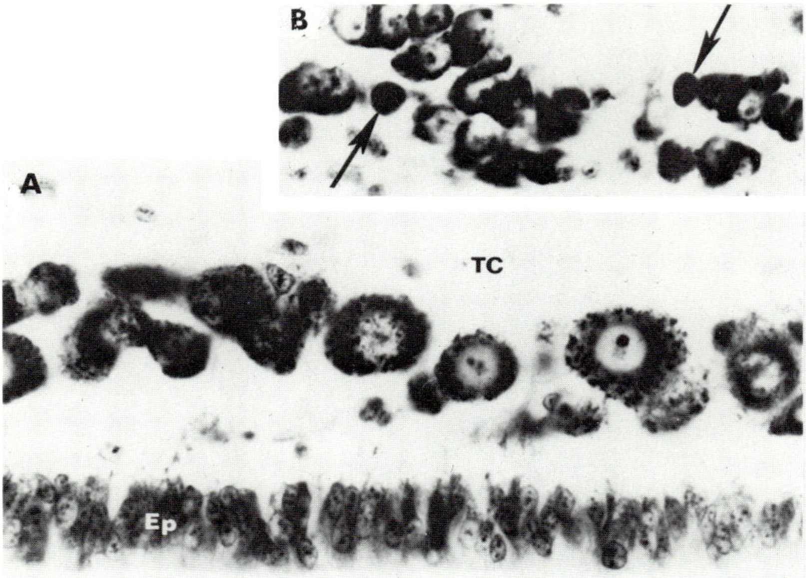

Fig. 6 A - To show the distinctive appearance of the cells of the mesencephalic nucleus of V in a 17-day-old chick (X540). TC: tectal commissure; Ep: ependyma. B - During the period of maximum cell loss in the nucleus a number of frankly degenerating neurons can be seen. Two such neurons are indicated by the arrows in this photomicrograph of a group of cells in the medial portion of the nucleus in an 11-day embryo (X410). (From Rogers and Cowan, 1973.)

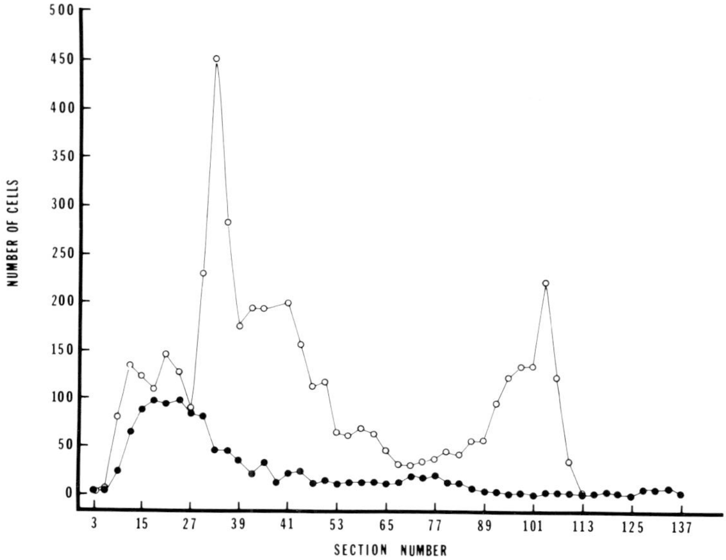

Fig. 7 In embryos up to the 9th day of incubation there are two peaks in the distribution of cells in the mesencephalic nucleus of V - one near its rostral pole and a second at its caudal end as this plot of the number of cells at successive rostrocaudal levels throughout the nucleus shows (open circles). After the cell loss that occurs between the 9th and 13th days of incubation, there is a general reduction in cell number throughout the nucleus (including its rostral pole) but the peak at the caudal end of the nucleus is completely eliminated (solid circles).

NEURONAL DEGENERATION IN AGING MAMMALS

Kalidas Nandy, M.D., Ph.D.

Department of Anatomy
Emory University
Atlanta, Georgia 30322

It is well known that when neurons are lost in mammals they are not replaced by division of the remaining cells. The loss of nerve cells is one of the most consistent changes in the brain of aging mammals. Ellis (1920) found a consistent decrease with age in the number of Purkinje cells per unit area of the cerebellum of adult humans (who were dying of causes thought unlikely to have a direct effect on brain cells). The cell density in the cerebral cortex of humans ranging in age from newborn to 95 years was studied by Brody (1955) who also reported a reduction in cell number with age in all cortical layers, with the greatest decrease occurring in the superior temporal gyrus and the area striata. Eckerstrom (1958) and Constanzo and Cognasso (1961) reported an increase in the γ-globulin fractions in the human serum with age. An age-related increase in auto-antibodies was also noted in aging mammals by Walford (1961) and Walford and Hildemann (1964) who suggested that these substances reflected changes in the immune mechanism. Amyloid lesions have been demonstrated in the brain parenchyma in older human subjects and it has been suggested that these materials resulted from auto-immune reactions (Walford and Sjaarda, 1964; Schwartz, 1965). An auto-immune theory of aging was proposed by Burnet (1959) and later by Comfort (1963) who suggested that a small number of immunologically competent cells might mutate in such a fashion as to lose tolerance to their "host's" antigens and subsequently give rise to a clone of cells producing antibodies which might result in death or damage to a large number of cells. In the present study, an attempt has been made to determine the role of immunological disturbance as a possible cause of neuronal degeneration in aging mammals.

C57 BL/6 female inbred mice of different ages (newborn to 30 months) were used in this study (Storer, 1966). Animals were kept in an environmental chamber with constant control of temperature (70-75°) and humidity (50-60%) and were fed on Purina mouse chow.

Anti-mouse rabbit γ-globulin (Chapel Laboratories, Downingtown, Pa.) was fractionated by means of sodium sulfate precipitation and dialysis against 0.02M phosphate buffer at pH 5.4 (Fritz et al., 1969). The final supernatant solution containing rabbit γ-globulin was conjugated with fluorescein isothiocynate (FITC) (BBL Division, Bio-Quest, Inc.) by the dialysis method of Clark and Shepard (1963).

A thorough intravascular perfusion was carried out by injecting phosphate-buffered saline (PBS, pH 7.1) into the left ventricle and letting the washed fluid out through the cut right atrium. The brains were then removed and frozen sections (10 μ) were cut in a cryostat. The sections were then fixed with 95% ethanol, washed with PBS and incubated at 37° C with fluorescein-labeled anti-mouse γ-globulin directly. Some sections were pretreated either with serum of a young or old mouse or its different protein fractions (albumin, α-, β- and γ-globulins) prior to incubation with FITC-labeled anti-mouse γ-globulin. The sections were then washed, mounted under a coverslip with glycerol-borate buffered saline solution (pH 8.1) and examined by ultraviolet microscopy.

Sera from old or young mice were injected directly into one cerebral hemisphere in either young or old mice using a 25 gauge needle and the contralateral hemisphere was injected with phosphate buffered saline (pH 7.1) as a control. The blood-brain barrier was damaged in heparinized animals by inserting a metal probe, chilled with dry ice (-70° C), into one cerebral hemisphere in old and young mice according to the method described by Bakay (1955). Animals were sacrificed 6-96 hours after the injury and coronal sections of the brain including both hemispheres were cut and treated by the above method.

Control tests for non-specific fluorescent staining of anti-mouse γ-globulin were carried out by absorption of anti-mouse γ-globulin with normal mouse serum prior to incubation and treatment of mouse brain sections with fluorescein-labeled normal rabbit globulin.

Four mice each from different age categories (newborn to 30 months) were tested for the presence of brain-reactive antibodies (BRA) in their sera by immunofluorescence method, and the percentage of cells in the brain sections showing positive reaction, when pretreated with their own sera prior to incubation with FITC-labeled anti-mouse γ-globulin, was calculated. Animals of the same age, sex, inbred strain and maintained in the same environment were used as controls.

Under nembutal anesthesia, the right sciatic nerve was cut and avulsed in 40 young (6 weeks) and 40 old (24 months) mice and three mice from each category were then sacrificed at different intervals following the operation (1, 3, 7, 14, 21, 28, 35, 42, 56, 70, 91, 120 days). The animals were perfused with phosphate-buffered saline (PBS) (pH 7.1) and two pieces of spinal cords (L_4-S_3 segments) were dissected out and frozen immediately in dry ice (at -70° C). Serial sections, ten μ thick, were cut in a cryostat and three successive sections, after every ten sections, were studied by histological and histochemical methods. Sections were fixed in 95% ethanol for histological staining and fresh frozen sections without fixation were mostly used for histochemical study of enzymes. The ventral horn neurons of the unaffected side of the spinal cord served as controls for the changes observed in the damaged side. The changes in the neurons damaged by cutting the sciatic nerve were compared with those in the degenerating neurons of old mice without experimental injury under a comparison microscope. Sections were stained with toluidine blue or Harris's hematoxylin and eosin to study morphological evidence of degeneration of the neurons. Sections were also stained by periodic acid-Schiff and counterstained by toluidine blue to visualize lipofuscin pigment in the degenerating neurons. The neuroglia were demonstrated by the ammoniacal silver carbonate method of Weil and Davenport (Culling, 1963). A number of enzymes, such as succinate and glucose-6-phosphate dehydrogenase (nitro BT method), acid phosphatase (napthal AS-BI method), adenosine triphosphatase (lead method), thiamine pyrophosphatase (lead method), and specific cholinesterase (acetylthiocholine iodide method), were studied by histochemical methods. Control tests were carried out by omitting the substrate in the incubation media and by using specific inhibitors for enzymes, whenever possible.

The possible migration of γ-globulin across BBB has been studied in 40 female (2-3 months old) C57 BL/6 mice using ^{125}I-labeled γ-globulin. γ-globulin was fractionated from the serum of 30-month-old mice and was labeled with ^{125}I by dialysis method. 10μc of ^{125}I-γ-globulin (0.3 mg of solution) was injected intraperitoneally into each animal. Then 0.1 ml of blood was drawn from the heart of each animal, under nembutal anesthesia, prior to sacrifice. At least three animals were sacrificed at different time intervals (6, 12, 18, 24, 36, 48, 72, 96, 120 hours) after the administration of the isotope. The animals were thoroughly perfused intravascularly with PBS and the ventricles of the brain were perfused with the same fluid by injecting the fluid into the two lateral ventricles and draining it out through the cut brain stem. The brain, including brain stem and cerebellum, liver, kidney, adrenal, heart, quadriceps femoris muscle, spleen, and thyroid were dissected out and weighed. The samples of blood (0.1 ml), pieces of organs (cerebrum, cerebellum, hypothalamus,heart, liver, adrenal, spleen, kidney, and skeletal muscle (10 mg each)) from each animal were placed in the glass tubes for γ-counting and were stored at -60° C until ready for use. All samples, the total dose of isotope in a tube, an empty tube (for background count) and the samples of blood and organs from two uninjected mice (control) were counted in a γ-counter (Packard) for ten minutes or 10,000 counts. The background count was subtracted from other counts before analysis of the data.

The antigen-antibody reaction was indicated by a bright greenish fluorescence mainly located either on the cell wall or in the nucleus of the nerve cells. Negative results, on the other hand, were indicated by a dark field without any greenish fluorescence except in cases of brain sections of old mice where orange-yellow autofluorescence of lipofuscin pigment was seen in the cytoplasm of the neurons.

When sections of brains of both young and old mice were first treated directly with sera from old mice and then incubated with FITC-labeled anti-mouse γ-globulin, specific fluorescence was observed in the neurons of both groups (Figs. 1, 2). When sections of brain of young and old mice were treated with fluorescein-labeled anti-mouse γ-globulin, no consistent specific staining was noted in the neurons. No specific reaction was observed in the neurons of young and old animals when serum from young mice was used in place of the old. When three different protein fractions of old mouse serum (albumin, β-globulin, and γ-globulin) were used in place of the serum of old mice, only the γ-globulin fractions gave typical fluorescence in the neurons (Fig. 3). It, therefore, appeared that antibody γ-globulin, which reacted with neurons, was present in sera of old mice but not in the young, and reacted with nerve cells of both young and old mice equally.

When the serum of old mice was injected directly into one cerebral hemisphere of old or young mice and frozen sections of the brain were treated with FITC-labeled anti-mouse γ-globulin, fluorescent staining was noted in a large number of neurons surrounding the area of injection in all mice (Fig. 4). No reaction was noted in the contralateral hemisphere or when the sera from young mice was injected. Damage to the blood-brain barrier by mechanical injury to one cerebral hemisphere in old mice resulted in a similar antigen-antibody reaction in the cells around the injured area (Fig. 5) and none in the contralateral hemisphere (Fig. 6). The same procedure in the brains of young mice did not show any specific reaction in the neurons.

Morphological evidence of degeneration was looked for in the neurons showing antigen-antibody reaction in old animals with damaged blood-brain barriers. Serial coronal sections of cerebrum of both groups of animals were alternately treated with FITC-labeled anti-mouse γ-globulin or stained with toluidine blue. It appears that 25% or more of the cells showing positive fluorescent staining also exhibited morphological evidence of degeneration (Fig. 7). Although some cells were injured directly by the operative procedure or vascular damage, the number of cells showing antigen-antibody reaction were far more numerous than this group. The degenerative changes were usually noticeable within 24-72 hours after the intracerebral injection of serum of old mice or the damage to the blood-brain barrier in old animals. The neurons of contralateral hemisphere and the control sections were mostly negative except for occasional degenerating cells in the brain of old animals.

When the brain-sections of mice of different ages were pretreated with their serum prior to incubation with FITC-labeled anti-mouse γ-globulin, a positive reaction was always noted if the serum contained BRA. The reaction was negative with serum from six months or younger mice and was consistently positive when serum from animals 15 months or older was used. The presence of specific antibodies was noted in serum of two out of four and three out of four in 9- and 12-month-old animals respectively. When the sections were treated with sera in different dilutions from mice of various ages, the dilution at which the fluorescence was completely eliminated increased progressively with the age of the animals (Fig. 11). A progressive increase in the number of cells showing specific greenish fluorescence in the brain sections was consistently observed when undiluted sera from mice of increasing age was used.

After the sciatic nerve of one side was cut, neurons located in the anterior and lateral parts of ventral horn of the same side showed signs of degeneration in both young and old mice within a week. The early changes included swelling of the cell body, hyperchromasia and eccentric position of the nucleus and dispersion and reduced basophilia of the Nissl substance in the cytoplasm. The degenerative changes in some cells lasted as long as three months when these cells were completely removed. About 3-4 weeks following the injury the cells, as a whole, appeared distorted, shrunken, the nucleus became lobulated or broken, the nucleoli looked pale and, finally, the cells became fragmented. The sequence of degenerative changes observed in the experimentally injured neurons were not seen in dying neurons in old animals without experimental injury. Distinct chromatolytic changes were not seen in neurons of these animals and the degenerating neurons were mostly identified by shrinkage and distortion of the cells and intense hyperchromasia of the nuclei with very little surrounding cytoplasm and, finally, fragmentation of the nuclei and the cell bodies.

An interesting type of glial reaction was observed around degenerating neurons in old animals without experimental injury. Neuroglial cells were seen surrounding dying neurons as well as some without any morphological evidence of degeneration in the brain of old mice (Fig.8). On the other hand, glial cells were mostly found around experimentally injured neurons with severe morphological degenerative changes in both young and old mice (Fig. 9). The nature of the glial cells and the precise significance of their appearance are not clear in this study. Lipofuscin pigment was demonstrated in the degenerating neurons, in both cases, in old mice by staining techniques used and often appeared to be the last remnant of the cells to be removed.

The reaction for succinate dehydrogenase was mostly located in the form of granules in the cytoplasm of the neurons and appeared to be progressively reduced starting as early as 7 days in the injured neurons in both young and old mice. In some cells, the trend changed after three weeks and the activity returned to normal within 63-91 days in both age groups. A progressive reduction of the enzyme activity was consistently seen in degenerating neurons without experimental injury in old animals and a reversal of this trend was not seen. The activity of glucose-6-phosphate dehydrogenase in neurons with cut axons differed from that in neurons in old mice without experimental injury. While progressive reduction of the enzyme was noted in the neurons of the latter group, an initial increase within 5-10 days followed by progressive decline was seen in the former. A progressive increase in acid phosphatase activity was found in all degenerating neurons in both age groups until the cells were broken down (Fig. 10), when the activity markedly declined. A progressive reduction of thiamine pyrophosphatase activity with a breakdown of the network pattern (i.e., retisolution) was noted in the cytoplasm of all degenerating neurons in different groups. The activities of both specific cholinesterase and adenosine triphosphatase appeared to be progressively reduced in degenerating neurons of both groups of animals.

The possible migration of γ-globulin across BBB in young mice has also been studied. A high level of radioactivity was observed in blood samples within 6 hours and the activity declined rapidly to almost 10% by 120 hours (Fig. 12). The activity of the isotope in the cerebrum and the cerebellum slowly increased from 6 hours to 24 hours and thereafter slowly declined by 120 hours. It was rather interesting to note that the highest activity in the brain samples was observed within 24 hours and only 40% of the activity was retained at 120 hours after the administration. While a low level of radioactivity was noted consistently in the brain tissue in all animals, the hypothalamus showed a relatively higher concentration of the isotope than the samples of cerebrum and cerebellum (Fig. 13).

An electrophoretic study on the extracted γ-globulin from blood samples and cerebral cortex was carried out on samples of blood and brain of two mice, and it was noted that 90% of the activity migrated at the same speed as the γ-globulin peak of the simultaneously tested original radio-globulin. It was assumed that the radioactivity counted in the tissues is still bound to the γ-globulin and not free or even bound to some other compound. A thorough perfusion of the blood vessels and ventricles of the brain has also been carried out, and it is assumed that counts in the brain tissues is due to the presence of γ-globulin in the neural tissue rather than in cerebrospinal fluid (CSF) or blood vessels.

Although in this study the γ-globulin binding fraction appears to be an antibody against neurons, an unequivocal statement cannot be made about this without such specific tests as precipitin, complement fixation, hemagglutination, etc. (Threatt *et al.*, 1971). The fact that little γ-globulin was associated with neurons of apparently healthy old mice, even though there were "anti-neuron" antibodies in their sera, might indicate presence of some barrier mechanism which allowed these antibodies to cross from the peripheral circulation into the brain at a very slow rate. The possible migration of γ-globulin into brain tissue of young $C_{57}BL/6$ mice has also been studied in our laboratory. It appears that the blood-brain barrier largely prevents the migration of circulating γ-globulin into the neural tissue and only a small quantity reaches the brain tissue. The rate of penetration increased during 6-24 hours and thereafter declined slowly as compared to the rate of decline in the blood. The permeability of the blood-brain barrier to various serum proteins, including γ-globulins, was also studied in cats using ^{131}I-labeled γ-globulin by a number of investigators who noted a slow rate of exchange of γ-globulin between blood, brain and cerebrospinal fluid under normal circumstances (Hochwald and Wallenstein, 1967; Bartin, 1960; Clausen, 1960; Day *et al.*, 1967).

The present study indicates that there is a progressive increase in the accumulation of BRA in the serum of $C_{57}BL/6$ mice as a function of age (Nandy, 1972a). Observations on increased concentration of immuno-globulin with advancing age have been made by a number of investigators (Karel et al., 1956; Eckerstrom, 1958; Constanzo and Cognasso, 1961; Walford, 1961; Nocker and Bemm, 1956; Parfenjev and Whitney, 1952). Age-related increases in strain-specific antibodies, such as rheumatoid factor in serum of apparently healthy humans, have been demonstrated (Kunkel, 1964). Antinuclear antibodies have been observed with increased incidence in older humans and in 15% of C57BL/6 mice (Kunkel, 1964). An increase in thyroid auto-antibodies with age was reported by Goodman, et al. (1963) based upon a study of 1,000 individuals including 396 schizophrenics.

The question as to whether the production of such antibodies is due to stimulation of the immune mechanism of the mice by microbial agents or is a result of auto-stimulation of the animals' own immune system has also been studied by using germ-free mice in our laboratory. Although an unequivocal statement cannot be made from this study, the evidence probably indicated that BRA found in the serum of old mice was produced as a result of stimulation of the immune system by the animals' own brain tissue, rather than by exogenous microbial agents (Nandy, 1972c).

A comparative study has also been made between the process of degeneration in neurons produced by severe axonal injury in the spinal cord of young and old mice and of aging mice without experimental injury. Although the cause of degeneration of neurons in aging animals is not clear in this study, it appears that these neurons mostly show signs of severe morphological degeneration without showing any evidence of regeneration. When the BBB was damaged in one cerebral hemisphere of old mice, serial sections of the brain showed antigen-antibody reaction by immuno-fluorescence method and evidence of cell damage by toluidine blue stain in a large number of cells in identical locations. Similar observations were made when sections stained by the immuno-fluorescent method were counterstained with toluidine blue. Specific fluorescence was noted only in occasional cells in the contralateral hemisphere, and these might represent the normally degenerating neurons in old animals. It appears that the degenerative changes observed in neurons of aging mice without experimental injury differed from those induced by axonal injury and may at least partly be due to an immunological reaction of neurons with brain-reactive antibodies present in the serum of old mice (Nandy, 1972b).

The role of such antibodies in neuronal degeneration in old animals is not clear in this study. The likely possibilities are that the antibody in the presence of complement might exert a cytotoxic effect upon the neurons, or the antigen-antibody reaction in the neurons, even in minute quantities, might attract the microglia toward the neurons leading to their destruction. Neuroglia have been found clustered both around neurons of old animals without demonstrable morphological signs of degeneration and also around markedly damaged neurons in cases of experimental injury. Andrew (1939) studied the process of neuronophagia by microglia in normal senile as well as severely starved mice and described the process to be essentially one of cytolysis of nerve cells. The cytotoxic effect of immune γ-globulin and complement on Krebs ascites tumor cells was studied electron microscopically by Green, _et al_. (1959), and they noted that exposure of cells to both antibody and complement resulted in severe damage to the cellular membranes, cytoplasmic matrix, mitochondria and endoplasmic reticulum. Goldberg, _et al_. (1959), on the other hand, noted a marked loss of free amino acid, RNA, and 90% of the intracellular potassium from cells treated with antibody and complement. These changes were less marked when antibody alone was used.

SUMMARY

The role of brain-reactive antibodies in the neuronal degeneration in aging mice has been studied. γ-globulin was seen to be associated with only a few nerve cells in brains of old mice when studied by immuno-fluorescence. When sections of brain of young and old mice were treated with serum from an old mouse prior to incubation with FITC-labeled anti-mouse rabbit γ-globulin, an antigen-antibody reaction was noted in a large number of cells in both groups. No specific fluorescence was noted when sera from young mice were used.

The relative change in the concentration of BRA in serum of C_{57}BL/6 mice with age has been studied, and it was observed that the onset of BRA in sera probably occurs at 6-15 months of age and thereafter increased progressively as a function of age.

The possible role of the BBB in the neuronal degeneration in aging was studied by damaging the blood-brain barrier in one cerebral hemisphere in old mice. A specific reaction, with evidence of degeneration, was noted in a large number of cells around the injured area. It appeared therefore that γ-globulin binding fraction (most likely antibody)against brain antigen is present in sera of old and not in young mice, and a barrier mechanism (possibly blood-brain barrier) plays an important role in separating the circulating antibodies from the brain cells. The possible migration of circulating γ-globulin into brain tissue has been investigated, and it was observed that the BBB prevents a large influx of γ-globulin at any given time and allows it to enter the brain at a rather slow rate. A comparative study indicated that neuronal degeneration in normally aging mice differs from the degeneration following axonal injury and is probably brought about by an immunological reaction of cells with neuron-reactive antibodies in the serum of old mice.

REFERENCES

Andrew, W. (1939). J. Comp. Neurol. 70, 413.

Bakay, L. (1955). Arch. Neurol. Psychiat. 73, 51.

Bartin, P. (1960). In "Analyse Imuno-Electrophoretique" (P. Grabar and P. Burtin, eds.), pp. 245-252, Masson et Cie, Paris.

Brody, H. (1955). J. Comp. Neurol. 102, 511.

Burnet, M. (1959). Brit. Med. J. 2, 720.

Clark, H.F. and Shepard, C.C. (1963). Virology 20, 642.

Clausen, J. (1960). World Neurol. 1, 479.

Comfort, A. (1963). Lancet 2, 138.

Constanzo, F. and Cognasso, P. (1961). Acta Gerontol. 11, 127.

Culling, C.F.A. (1963). "Handbook of Histopathological Techniques." Butterworth, Washington.

Day, E.D., Rigsbee, L., Wilkins, R. and Mahaley, M.S., Jr. (1967). J. Immunol. 98, 62.

Eckerstrom, S.F. (1958). Geriatrics 13, 744.

Ellis, R.S. (1920). J. Comp. Neurol. 32, 1.

Fritz, R.B., Langlois, A.J. and Beard, J.W. (1969). Virology 4, 372.

Goldberg, B., Burton, C. and Green, H. (1959). J. Exp. Med. 109, 505.

Goodman, H., Rosenblatt, M., Gottlieb, J.S., Miller, J.

and Chen, C.H. (1963). Arch. Gen. Psychiat. 8, 518.
Green, H., Gleischer, R.A., Barrow, P. and Goldberg, B. (1959). J. Exp. Med. 109, 511.
Hochwald, G.M. and Wallenstein, M.C. (1967). Exp. Neurol. 19, 115.
Karel, J.L., Wilder, V.M. and Beber, M. (1956). J. Am. Geriat. Soc. 4, 667.
Kunkel, H.G. (1964). Fed. Proc. 23, 623.
Nandy, K. (1972a). J. Gerontol. 27, 173.
Nandy, K. (1972b). Exp. Gerontol. 7, 303.
Nandy, K. (1972c). Mech. Age. Dev. 1, 133.
Nocker, J. and Bemm, H. (1956). Z. Alternsforsch. 9, 328.
Parfentjev, I.A. and Whitney, L.F. (1952). J. Gerontol. 7, 490.
Schwartz, P. (1965). Trans. N. Y. Acad. Sci. II, 27, 393.
Storer, J.B. (1966). J. Gerontol. 21, 404.
Threatt, J., Nandy, K. and Fritz, R. (1971). J. Gerontol. 26, 316.
Walford, R.L. (1961). In "Advances in Gerontological Research" (B.L. Strehler, ed.), pp. 159-204, Academic Press, New York.
Walford, R.L. and Sjaarda, J.R. (1964). J. Gerontol. 19,57.
Walford, R.L. and Hildemann, W.H. (1964). Transplantation 2, 87.

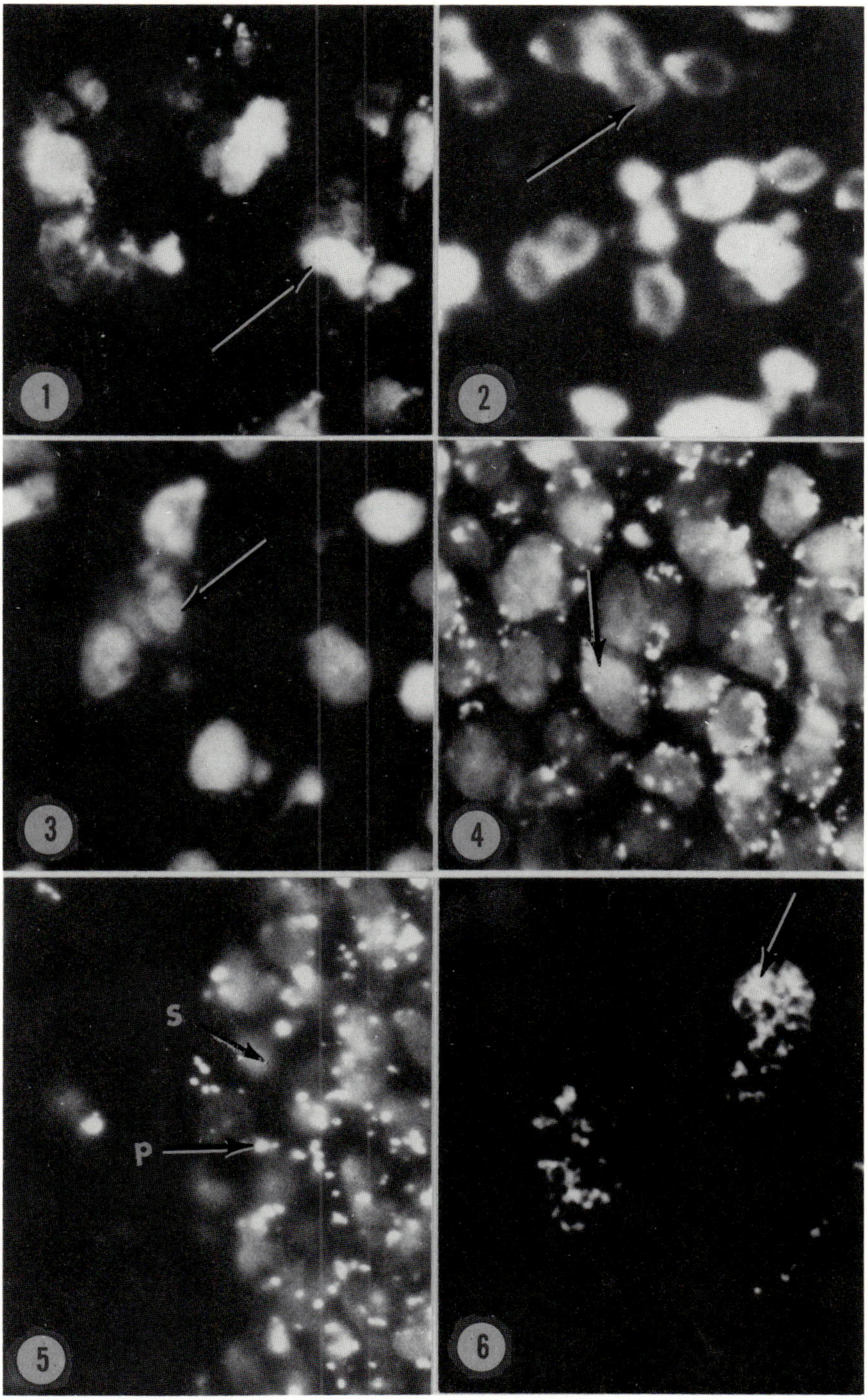

Captions for Plate I on following page

Plate I

Fig. 1 Section (10μ) of cerebrum of an old mouse (18 months). The section was treated with serum of an old mouse prior to incubation with FITC-labeled anti-mouse γ-globulin. Note the strong specific fluorescence in the neurons due to antigen-antibody reaction (arrow). x 675

Fig. 2 Section (10μ) of brain of a young mouse (3 months). Sections were pretreated with serum of an old mouse prior to incubation with fluorescein-labeled anti-mouse γ-globulin. Note the strong specific fluorescence in the cell wall (arrow). x 675

Fig. 3 Same as Fig. 2 except that the serum of an old mouse was replaced by its γ-globulin fraction. Note the specific reaction (arrow) in the neurons. x 675

Fig. 4 Section of the cerebrum of an old mouse (18 months). Note the specific fluorescence (arrow) in the neurons around the area of intracerebral injection of serum from an old mouse (18 months). Note also the autofluorescence of granular lipofuscin. x 675

Fig. 5 Section of cerebrum of an old mouse (18 months). Note the specific fluorescence (S) in the neurons around the area of damage to the blood-brain barrier in one cerebral hemisphere. Also note the autofluorescence of lipofuscin (P). x 675

Fig. 6 Section of contralateral cerebral hemisphere in same animal as in Fig. 5. Note the absence of specific staining in the neurons. Also note the autofluorescence of lipofuscin (arrows) in the cytoplasm. x 675

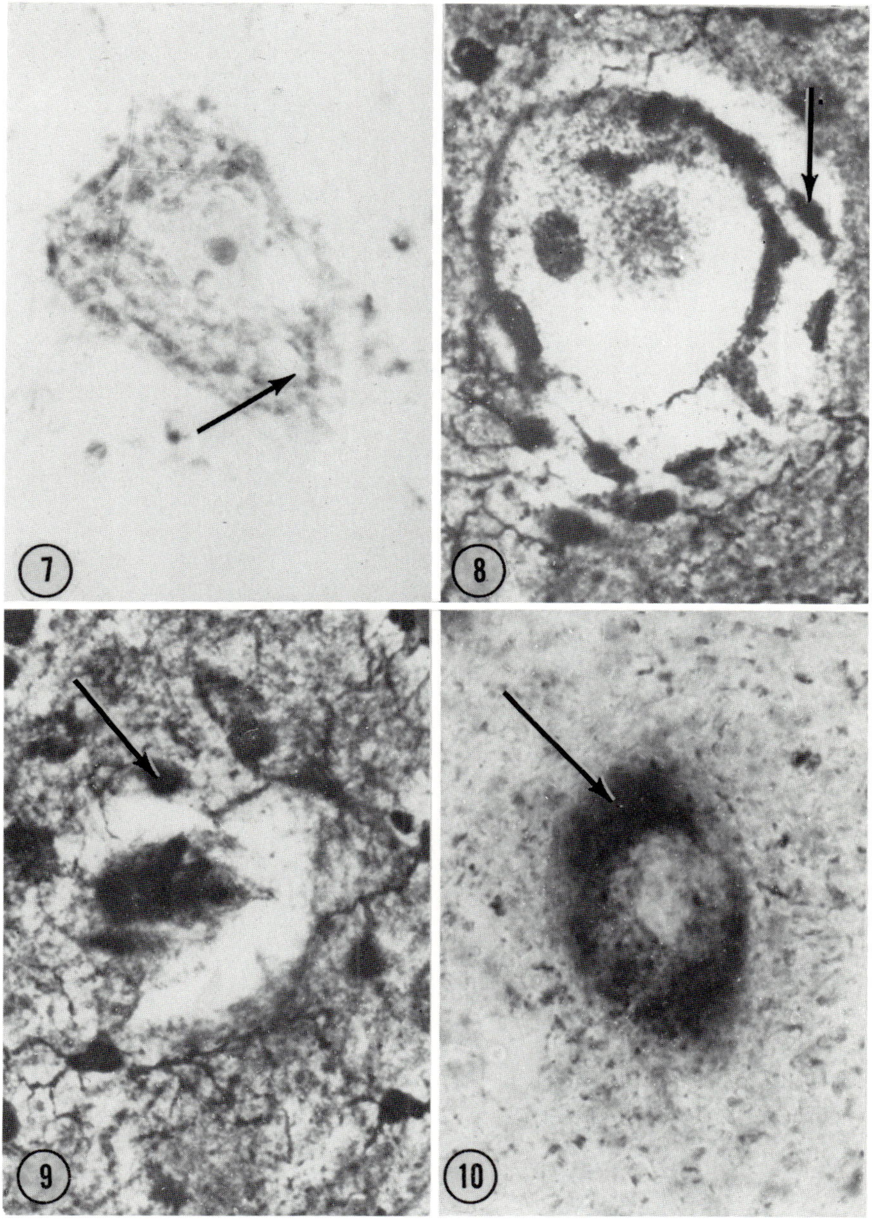

Captions for Plate II on following page

Plate II

Fig. 7 Serial section of the brain as in Fig. 5 stained with toluidine blue. Note the severe chromatolysis in the cytoplasm (arrow) of the neuron near the damaged BBB.

Fig. 8 Section of cerebral cortex from a 30-month-old mouse stained by ammoniacal silver carbonate method (Weil-Davenport). Note that the apparently normal neuron is surrounded by neuroglia (arrow). x 855

Fig. 9 Section of spinal cord of 6-month-old mouse with cut sciatic nerve. Note the severely damaged neuron in the ventral horn surrounded by neuroglia. x 855

Fig. 10 Pyramidal cell of cerebral cortex undergoing degeneration near the area of damage to BBB in an 18-month-old mouse. Note the increased reaction (arrow) of acid phosphatase in the cytoplasm of a neuron. x 855

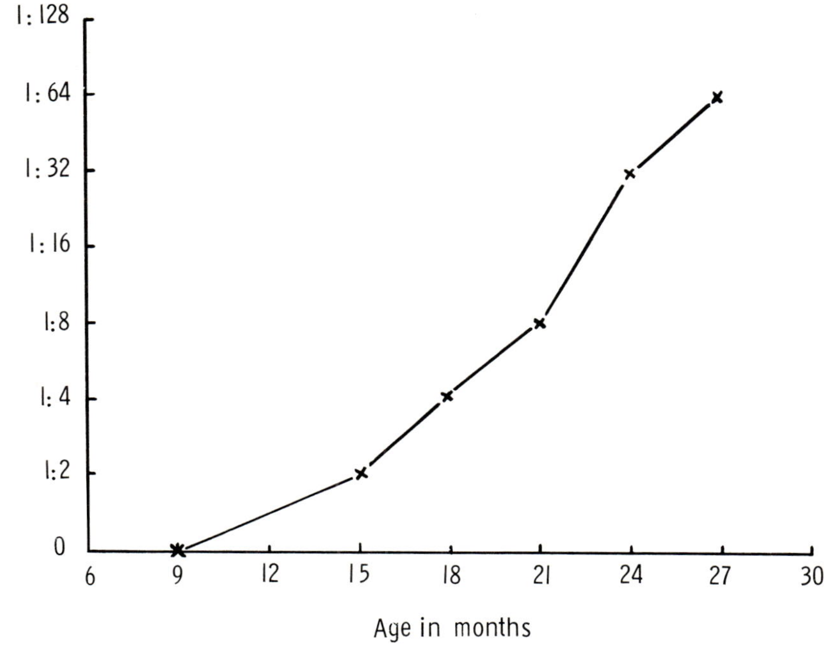

Fig. 11 The points of extinction of specific fluorescence in neurons when sections of cerebral cortex were treated with sera in different dilutions from mice of various age groups. Note that the dilution required to eliminate fluorescence increased progressively with the age of the mice.

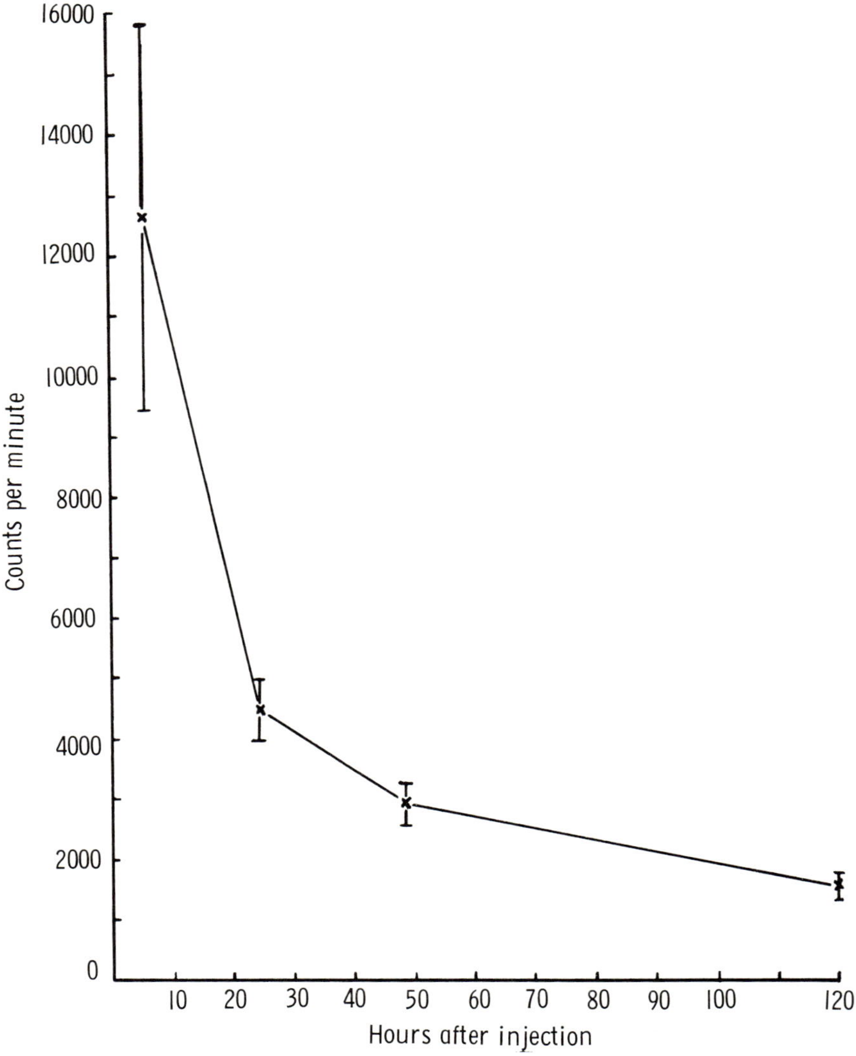

Fig. 12 Levels of radioactivity in blood at different time intervals after intraperitoneal injection of ^{125}I-labeled γ-globulin.

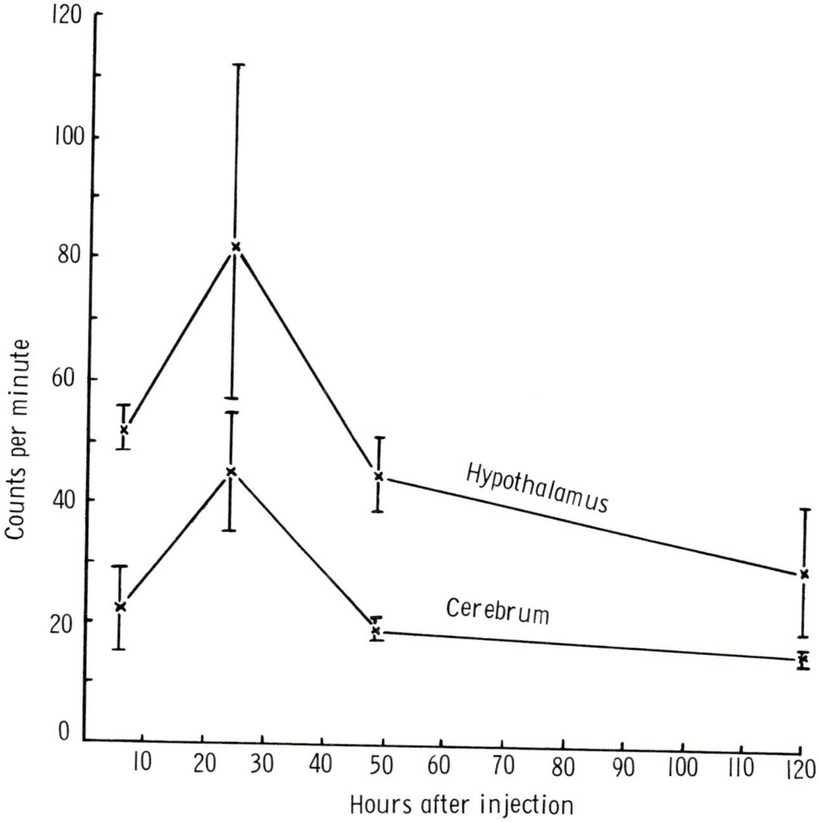

Fig. 13 Levels of radioactivity in cerebrum and hypothalamus at different time intervals after intraperitoneal injection of ^{125}I-labeled γ-globulin.

SELECTED CHANGES IN THE DEVELOPING POSTNATAL RAT BRAIN[1]

Donald H. Ford

Department of Anatomy
Downstate Medical Center
Brooklyn, New York

Developmental changes in the brains of mammals just before birth and in the early postnatal period are most dramatic, both morphologically and biochemically. The time and rate at which these changes occur vary considerably with the species studied (Himwich, in press). In the rat, brain weight at birth is approximately 15% of the adult level, which is attained at about 120 days of age (Fig. 1). A similar growth curve for rat brain has been reported by de Souza and Dobbing (1971) using absolute weights (note that man and monkey show comparable growth curves when plotted against a series of arbitrary age equivalents). In the first 20 days after birth, neurons have been observed to grow rapidly, increasing in weight and volume (Ford and Cohan, 1968; Gregory and Ford, 1970) as well as in the extent of their processes (Eayrs and Goodhead, 1959; Morest, 1969; Schadé and Meeter, 1963). Synaptic connections are established (Aghajanian and Bloom, 1967) and mitochondrial profiles increase in number (Pysh, 1970). This, of course, could be due as much to an increase in cells (mainly glia) as to an increase in the number per cell. The increase in mitochondrial volume may be related to the specific role played by mitochondria in neonatal brain tissue in protein synthesis (Sokoloff and Roberts, 1971) as well as to

[1]Supported in part by a U.S. Public Health Service NIH Grant NB-04568-08 and in part by a U.S. Public Health Service training grant to the Department of Anatomy (5TIG M 379-09) and in part by a research contract from the Physiology Branch of the Office of Naval Research (NONR 4018 (00)).

cellular respiration. Enzymes concerned with the synthesis of transmitter substance increase in activity (Coyle and Axelrod, 1972a, b) as do the levels of norepinephrine and seratonin (Hyyppä, 1971). Dopamine shows essentially no change in level per gram wet weight during this maturational period (Hyyppä, 1971), but should be reevaluated on a per neuron basis. During this same period, monoamine oxidase, a degradative enzyme of amines, shows an increase comparable to that observed for norepinephrine (Vaccari _et al._, 1972) (Fig. 2). Respiratory enzyme systems for anaerobic glycolysis become less significant as enzymes associated with aerobic glycolysis attain greater prominence. In the first four to five days, there is a marked gliogenesis (Brizzee _et al._, 1964) which is quickly followed by an increase in glial protein synthesis and finally myelinization (Schonbach _et al._, 1968). As these events are occurring, there is a decrease in brain water content (Soriero and Ford, 1971; de Souza and Dobbing, 1971; Vernadakis and Woodbury, 1962), which is paralleled by an increase in brain solids (Soriero and Ford, 1971, and in press). Potassium levels/kg wet weight increase (Vernadakis and Woodbury, 1962), while sodium and chloride levels decrease (de Souza and Dobbing, 1971; Vernadakis and Woodbury, 1962). There are, in addition, changes in the free brain nucleotides (Mandel and Edel-Harth, 1966) in which the adenine nucleotides show the most prominent increase, paralleling the increasing levels of energy metabolism in the maturing brain. Studies by Fish and Winick (1969) have also demonstrated an increase in DNA and RNA per mg of whole brain, reflecting the increase in total cell numbers, in cell size, and in the RNA content. The latter has been more specifically demonstrated in hippocampal neurons by Ringborg (1966), who observed a rapid increase in RNA from birth to adulthood and finally an appreciable loss in severe old age.

While the bulk of cell division occurring in the brain after birth may be related to the oligodendroglial cells, there is a significant increase in microneurons of the cerebellum, because a large part of the basket and stellate cells of the mature cerebellar cortex are derived by mitosis from granule cell of the external granule cell layer, after birth (Altman, 1969; Altman and Das, 1966; Angevine, 1965).

Without having discussed details, the foregoing

illustrate the tremendous morphological and biochemical changes occurring in the rat brain in the first 20 to 25 days after birth. The changes are of fundamental importance for the subsequent physiological activity of the brain. While other mammals, including man, may have different time tables for these events, there is little doubt that similar changes occur. What then should be almost self evident is that the brain, while undergoing differentiation and maturation may be more vulnerable to a variety of factors than in adulthood. As discussed by Dobbing (1968), there appears to be a period of particular vulnerability corresponding to the time of major development for a wide range of maturational or differentiational changes. Thus, micro- and macroneurogenesis, gliogenesis, myelinization, formation of specific proteins and enzyme systems do not occur simultaneously, but may overlap each other. Each may have a specific time for a "developmental spurt" when they are most vulnerable to numerous factors which may alter the milieu of the brain. Nutritional deficiencies (Balázs and Patel, in press; Smart and Dobbing, 1971a, b), hormonal dyscrasias (Balázs _et al._, 1968, 1969, 1971; Eayrs, 1964, 1968; Hamburgh, 1969; Pasquini _et al._, 1967; de Vellis _et al._, 1971; de Vellis and Inglish, in press), X-irradiation (Altman _et al._, 1968; Cohan and Ford, 1969; Cohan _et al._, 1969; Rugh, 1968; Schjeide _et al._, 1968; Valcana _et al._, 1972; Vernadakis and Timiras, 1963; Vernadakis _et al._, 1968) and experiential factors (Bennett _et al._, 1964a, b; Krech _et al._, 1966; Riege, 1971) and anoxia (Hicks _et al._, 1962) have all been shown to influence the developing brain.

Morphological Changes:

I would like to direct this discussion to certain morphological and biochemical changes which occur in the postnatal period which may be related and which may influence the interpretation of other parameters of maturation.

Growth of neurons in several species has been reported by Eayrs and Goodhead (1959), Ford and Cohan (1968), Fox, _et al._ (1966), Gregory and Ford (1970), Noback and Purpura (1961), Schadé and various co-workers (1960, 1961, 1962, 1963). These may be illustrated by measurements of cell volume and weight (Fig. 3), both of which increase rapidly in the early postnatal days. This is most marked in the ventral horn motoneurons of spinal cord, which also grow appreciably larger than do the pyramidal neurons of layer 5 (taken from the dorsum of the cortex at the level of the anterior commissure (motor and premotor cortex). In addition, the ventral horn neurons continue to grow in size beyond 24 days of immediate postnatal life, continuing on for several months, while the pyramidal cells commence to decrease in size. At this point, a significant difference in cell size develops between male and female animals. This decrease in pyramidal cell size was also noted by Brizzee and Jacobs (1959) in cells measured after the 20th postnatal day. However, the volumes they report are considerably smaller, which could be due to differences in the strain of rats studied as well as the formula used for determining volume. These changes in cell volume parallel very closely those reported for whole brain weight (Adlard and Dobbing, 1971; Clouet and Gaitonde, 1956; Mandel and Edel-Harth, 1966). As the nerve cell bodies enlarge, the extent and complexity of their processes also increases (Eayrs and Goodhead, 1959; Schadé and Baxter, 1960; Schadé and Meeter, 1963). This may be illustrated by examining the axonal density (Fig. 4) of the molecular layer (layer 1) of sensorimotor cortex wherein there is a rapid increase in the number of axons per unit volume within the first week, which actually exceeds the final adult density (Eayrs and Goodhead, 1959). Electron microscopically recognizable synapses (Fig. 4) also show a period of rapid formation postnatally (Aghajanian and Bloom, 1967). Unfortunately, the areas examined by the two groups are not comparable, leaving one to assume that these changes occur at comparable rates in different cortical areas.

Amino Acids and Protein:

Measurements of increases in neuronal weight and volume provide only a partial image of the morphological changes which occur postnatally. As the cells grow in size and increase the extent of their processes, they become widely dispersed. This reduces the volume of brain grey matter occupied by neuronal soma (Fig. 5). This is significant in relation to measurements of protein synthesis which appear to occur largely in neuronal soma, as determined by labeled amino acid incorporation studies

(Altman, 1964; Ford and Rhines, 1969, 1970a, b). Thus, if one were to assume that neurons of neonatal and adult rats were to synthesize protein at equivalent rates per unit weight or volume of cell, one would expect that the accumulation of a labeled amino acid into protein in the neonatal rats would be higher than in adults because the volume of grey matter occupied by soma is appreciably larger (20% at 7 days) in the spinal cord as compared to 10% at 6 weeks. (Neuronal soma also occupy about 10% of the volume of the cerebral grey.) Various neurochemical studies confirm the higher accumulation of amino acids into the protein of neonatal brain (Adams and Lim, 1966; Gelber _et al._, 1964; Lajtha, 1964; de Vellis _et al._, 1967; Yamagami _et al._, 1966) and generally attribute the difference between neonatal and adult brain to the relative ineffectiveness of the blood-brain barrier in young animals. This conclusion has persisted despite observations that accumulation of labeled amino acid in neonatal tissue is also higher than in adults when homogenates, brain slices or particulate fractions are studied (Johnson and Luttges, 1966; Murthy and Rappoport, 1965; Vahvelainen and Oja, 1969). This appears particularly clear from the data of Oja (1972) on rat brain homogenates (Table 1) wherein he analyzed the incorporation of phenylalanine, tyrosine and tryptophan into protein. The apparent increase in K_m with age indicates that there was a higher affinity of amino acids for protein synthesis in neonatal than in adult brain. Kinetically, this could be an important factor in the lower levels of incorporation of labeled amino acid into protein in adults, possibly related to a reduced requirement for protein synthesis in essentially non- or slowly-growing cells. The changes in the maximal velocity (V_{max}) of incorporation of amino acid were also higher in neonates, which could be due to several factors: 1) the more rapid exhaustion of energy sources (Oja, 1966) and 2) the greater instability of large mRNA-ribosome complexes (Zomzely _et al._, 1968) in adult brains. It should be pointed out that the interpretation of such data is complicated by many factors (see Oja, 1972) relating to the as yet incomplete information on the intracellular contents of enzymes and metabolic compartments. Finally, we contend that while the blood-brain barrier exerts a control over influx and efflux of amino acids between brain and blood, a significant percent of the difference in amino acid incorporation into brain protein between neonates and adults is associated with the percent of grey matter occupied by the cell bodies. The rate of growth of the neurons as well as such factors as the rapid proliferation of glia in the postnatal animal in relation to myelin synthesis, and those factors indicated by Oja (1972) are also of significance. Table 2 illustrates the changes in volume of spinal grey matter occupied by neuronal soma in relation to age, weights of motoneurons and the amount of ^{3}H-lysine accumulated per unit weight. Observations of Guroff and Udenfriend (1964) also suggest that the higher uptake of amino acids in neonatal brain are more due to metabolic determinants than to the degree of development of a barrier. A factor undoubtedly related to both the observations of Oja and Guroff is the recent findings that the concentration of total tRNA in the supernatant fraction of rat brain decreases during the postnatal maturational period (Barra _et al_., 1972). The tRNA for specific amino acids decreased for phenylalanine, lysine, proline, and valine, was essentially unchanged for glycine and increased for leucine, alanine and isoleucine. When the data was expressed in terms of pmole of a specific tRNA/g of brain, the total of all the tRNAs showed a decrease between 4 and 55 days of age. In view of the role of tRNA in protein synthesis, this decrease in activity with age appears of major significance in relation to the rate of protein synthesis in neonates versus adults.

A further aspect of protein synthesis in rat brain during development pertains to a sex difference in the degree of accumulation of labeled amino acid into protein (Kartzinel _et al_., 1971). Accumulation of ^{3}H-lysine/gm of protein following intravenous injection of labeled amino acid decreased in both male and female brains between 1, 3 and 5 weeks of age in the expected manner (Fig. 6). However, it was noted that there was a significantly higher incorporation in male brain protein in animals killed 2 hours after injection at one week of age. At 3 weeks, there were no differences, while by 5 weeks of age, the levels of amino acid incorporation were significantly higher in males at all time intervals after injection.

During this same period, the labeling of plasma protein by ^{3}H-lysine increased markedly, but demonstrated no sex differences. In view of the fact that this experiment (like many others) involved providing a single pulse injection of labeled amino acid, the very marked increase in labeling of plasma proteins between 1 and 3 weeks of age may be quite significant in relation to the labeling of brain protein. Since the dose of amino acid per gram of rat is the same at all ages, the increased rapid labeling of plasma proteins should markedly reduce the levels of free amino acids available in the plasma. Inasmuch as it is the free amino acids which are available for transport into brain (Lajtha, 1964), the amount of ^{3}H-lysine which could become incorporated into the brains of the older animals should then be proportionally reduced. Thus, there would be an apparent reduction in protein synthesis which would in actuality be unrelated to barriers, tRNAs, growth, etc., but would be related to the experimental design which would in no way duplicate the normal state of a relatively constant level of the amino acid being available for transport into the brain.

RNA:

Studies on the levels of RNA (essentially ribosomal) in neonatal male and female brains revealed age and sex differences between 1-, 3- and 5-week-old animals (Fig. 7) in limbic and non-limbic structures (Soriero and Ford, 1971). There was a significant decrease in the concentration of RNA/μg of protein between 1 and 3 weeks of age in the hippocampus, hypothalamus, occipital cortex and cerebellar vermis. In addition, the vermis showed a continued reduction in RNA in the fifth week, which was not demonstrated by the other regions of brain. Significant sex differences in RNA concentration were observed in the hippocampus, hypothalamus and vermis at the points indicated by the + symbol. An evaluation of the adenine + uracil/guanine + cytosine ratio (^{E}260 mu/^{E}280) (Fig. 8) indicated a decrease in the ratio between 1 and 3 weeks of age which was significant for all tissues but the vermis. This was followed by an increase of somewhat greater magnitude between 3 and 5 weeks, which was also significant for all tissues but the vermis. However, the vermis did show an overall increase in the above ratio between 1 and 5 weeks of age. A sex difference was also noted in this ratio at 1 week of age in the hypothalamus. Since an A+U/G+C ratio of greater than one would represent mainly nuclear RNA, these ratios suggest that the cells being measured have a relatively large amount of nucleoplasm in relation to the cytoplasm. The higher ratios observed in the female hypothalamus would seem to be consistent with the observation that nuclear volumes of neurons of the preoptic area and the hypothalamic ventromedian nucleus are larger in fetal, neonatal and mature females (Döerner and Staudt, 1969). These differences in RNA between males and females suggest an inherent sex difference in biochemical maturation of the CNS.

Thyroid Hormone:

One of the factors known to influence protein synthesis and development of the brain is thyroid hormone (Klee and Sokoloff, 1964). This appears to be particularly true in the first 5 to 10 neonatal days (Sokoloff and Roberts, 1971). This leads us to consider the possibility of an age difference in thyroid hormone (^{131}I-triiodothyronine) accumulation in brain tissue (Bleecker *et al.*, 1971; Ford and Rhines, 1970c). The role of gender was also investigated.

^{131}I-triiodothyronine was injected intravenously into a series of rats 2, 4, 8 and 14 weeks of age and the accumulation of labeled hormone determined 1/2, 1, 2, 4 and 7 hours after injection. In both sexes there was a significant increase in hormone accumulation with increasing age in the cerebral grey matter between 1 and 8 weeks of age, with the females usually having higher values of accumulation (Fig. 9). This was then followed by a significant drop in accumulation in the 14-week-old animals in both sexes, with the females still maintaining a higher uptake than males. Significantly higher accumulations occurred in the 8- and 14-week-old female rats in cerebral grey matter, hypothalamus, thalamus, cerebellum and brain stem. From these observations, it would appear that triiodothyronine accumulation is lowest in the period when cell growth is most rapid and when the rate of protein synthesis is highest. This may be due to some specific relationship between thyroid hormone and protein synthesis, which is known to be facilitated in neonates by thyroxine (Sokoloff and Roberts, 1971). Furthermore, since the concentration of brain protein/gram dry weight is somewhat less in neonates, there would presumably be less thyroid hormone specific binding protein present. While this would permit more of the hormone to remain unbound, permitting its biological activity (Tata, 1964), it would also allow for a greater degree of degradation and loss through deiodination (Tata, 1964). Degradation and loss in neonates may also be further facilitated by the presence of an enzyme splitting the hormone at the ether bond (Cohan *et al.*, 1969) (Tables 3 and 4). Free iodide levels were extremely variable, but tended to be lower in the older animals. The iodide level is somewhat difficult to interpret, however, because of its rapid entry into blood. Thus, in neonates a lower lever of ^{131}I-activity was observed to be present in the brain as hormone than in more mature animals, while the levels of mono- and diiodotyrosine were higher than in the older animals. These changes were also reflected in the plasma wherein the hormonal levels were lower in the 1-week-old rats than at 4 weeks, while the iodinated tyrosines were higher at the younger age. Iodide levels in plasma at the various ages were not significantly different.

Examination of the triiodothyronine accumulation in the adenohypophyses of neonatal and young adult rats demonstrated more or less the same age and sex differences as were seen in the cerebral grey (Bleecker *et al.*, 1971), with some differences in the patterns of the curves suggesting differences in uptake, utilization or binding. Plasma levels of labeled hormone were essentially equivalent for both sexes, with greater age differences among the female group. Thus, the sex differences in hormone accumulation would seem to be inherent within the tissues and relate to such factors as transport, utilization, degradation, and binding.

Time and space do not permit a detailed listing and discussion of all the forms of maturation in the neonatal rat brain which occur in the short period just after birth. What has been presented are several lines of evidence indicating that there are changes in the morphological heterogeneity of the tissue and the rates at which growth occur at different ages which will influence measurements of protein synthesis and perhaps hormone accumulation which are unrelated to the blood-brain barrier. Our lack of understanding is further impeded by our lack of knowledge of what transpires between neurons and glia and of the effects of maturation on metabolic compartmentation. We might also ask, are there differences in amino acid pool size within neurons with changing age?; how does this relate to the levels of tRNA or other forms of RNA and eventually the synthesis of protein? Furthermore, what emerges from the various studies of the developing brain is that it is a tissue of extreme and changing heterogeneity during the early postnatal period. During this period the growth of cells and their processes, the maturation of enzyme systems and protein synthesis, and the accumulation and degradation of hormones are vulnerable to a wide variety of conditions varying from nutritional-hormonal states to the effects of experience and irradiation.

REFERENCES

Adams, D.H. and Lim, L. (1966). Biochem. J. 99, 261.

Adlard, B.P.F. and Dobbing, J. (1971). Brain Res. 28, 97.

Aghajanian, G.K. and Bloom, F.E. (1967). Brain Res. 6, 716.

Altman, J. (1964). In "Response of the Nervous System to Ionizing Radiation" (T.J. Haley and R.S. Snider, eds.), 2nd Ed., p. 336, Little, Brown & Co., Boston.

Altman, J. (1969). J. Comp. Neurol. 137, 433.

Altman, J. and Das, G.D. (1966). J. Comp. Neurol. 126, 337.

Altman, J., Anderson, W.J. and Wright, K.A. (1968). Exp. Neurol. 21, 69.

Angevine, J.B. (1965). Exp. Neurol. Suppl. 2, 1.

Balázs, R., Brooksbank, B.W.L., Davison, A.N., Eayrs, J.T. and Wilson, D.A. (1969). Brain Res. 15, 219.

Balázs, R., Kovacs, S., Teichgräber, P., Cocks, W.A., and Eayrs, J.T. (1968). J. Neurochem. 15, 1335.

Balázs, R., Kovacs, S., Cocks, W.A., Johnson, A.L. and Eayrs, J.T. (1971). Brain Res. 25, 555.

Balázs, R. and Patel, A.J. (1973). In "The Neurobiology of Maturation and Aging" (D.H. Ford, ed.), Elsevier, Amsterdam (in press).

Barra, H.S., Unates, L.E., Sayavedra, M.D. and Caputto, R. (1972). J. Neurochem. 19, 2289.

Bennett, E.L., Diamond, M.C., Krech, D. and Rosenzweig, M. R. (1964a). Science 146, 610.

Bennett, E.L., Krech, D. and Rosenzweig, M.R. (1964b). J. Comp. Physiol. Psychol. 57, 440.

Bleecker, M.L., Ford, D.H. and Rhines, R.K. (1971). In "Influence of Hormones on the Nervous System" (D.H. Ford, ed.), pp. 231-239, Karger AG, Basel.

Brizzee, K.R. and Jacobs, L.A. (1959). Acta Anat. 38, 291.

Brizzee, K.R., Vogt, J. and Kharetchko, X. (1964). In

"Growth and Maturation of the Brain" (D. Purpura and J.P. Schadé, eds.), Prog. Brain Res. 4, 325, Elsevier, Amsterdam.

Clouet, D.H. and Gaitonde, M.K. (1956). J. Neurochem. 1, 126.

Cohan, S.L. and Ford, D.H. (1969). Acta Neurol. Scandinav. 45, 53.

Cohan, S.L., Ford, D.H., Rhines, R.K. and Thompson, D. (1969). Acta Neurol. Scandinav. 45, 129.

Coyle, J.T. and Axelrod, J. (1972a). J. Neurochem. 19, 449.

Coyle, J.T. and Axelrod, J. (1972b). J. Neurochem. 19,1117.

DeSouza, S.W. and Dobbing, J. (1971). Exp. Neurol. 32, 431.

de Vellis, J. and Inglish, D. (1973). In "The Neurobiology of Maturation and Aging" (D.H. Ford, ed.), Elsevier, Amsterdam (in press).

de Vellis, J., Inglish, D., Cole, R. and Molson, J. (1971). In "Influence of Hormones on the Nervous System" (D.H. Ford, ed.), pp. 25-39, Karger, AG, Basel.

de Vellis, J., Schjeide, O.A. and Clemente, C.D. (1967). J. Neurochem. 14, 499.

Dobbing, J. (1968). In "Applied Neurochemistry" (A.N. Davison and J. Dobbing, eds.), pp. 287-316, Blackwells, Oxford.

Döerner, G. and Staudt, J. (1969). Neuroendocrinology 5, 103.

Eayrs, J.T. (1964). Animal Behavior 12, 195.

Eayrs, J.T. (1968). In "Endocrinology and Human Behavior" (R.P. Michael, ed.), pp. 239-255, Oxford University Press, London.

Eayrs, J.T. and Goodhead, B. (1959). J. Anat. 93, 385.

Fish, I. and Winick, M. (1969). Pediat. Res. 3, 407.

Ford, D.H. and Cohan, G. (1968). Acta Anat. 71, 311.

Ford, D.H. and Rhines, R.K. (1969). Acta Neurol. Scandinav. 45, 41.

Ford, D.H. and Rhines, R.K. (1970a). J. Neurol. Sci. 10, 179.

Ford, D.H. and Rhines, R.K. (1970b). J. Neurol. Sci. 10, 331.

Ford, D.H. and Rhines, R.K. (1970c). Brain Res. 21, 265.

Fox, M.W., Inman, O.R. and Himwich, W.A. (1966). J. Comp. Neurol. 127, 199.

Gelber, S., Cambell, P.L., Deikler, E.G. and Sokoloff, L. (1964). J. Neurochem. 11, 221.

Gregory, E. and Ford, D.H. (1970). Anat. Rec. 166, 310.

Guroff, G. and Udenfriend, S. (1964). In "The Developing Brain" (W.A. Himwich, ed.), Prog. Brain Res. 9, 187, Elsevier, Amsterdam.

Hamburgh, M. (1969). In "Current Topics in Developmental Biology" (A. Monroy and A.A. Moscona, eds.), Vol. 4, p. 109, Academic Press, New York.

Hicks, S.P., Cavanaugh, M.C. and O'Brien, E.D. (1962). Am. J. Pathol. 40, 615.

Himwich, W.A. (1973). In "The Neurobiology of Maturation and Aging" (D.H. Ford, ed.), Elsevier, Amsterdam (in press).

Hyyppä, M. (1971). Experientia 27, 336.

Johnson, T.C. and Luttges, M.W. (1966). J. Neurochem. 13, 545.

Kartzinel, R., Ford, D.H. and Rhines, R.K. (1971). In "Influence of Hormones on the Nervous System" (D.H. Ford, ed.), pp. 296-305, Karger AG, Basel.

Klee, C.B. and Sokoloff, L. (1964). J. Neurochem. 11, 709.

Krech, D., Rosenzweig, M.R. and Bennett, E.L. (1966). Physiol. Behavior 1, 99.

Lajtha, A. (1964). Intern. Rev. Neurobiol. 6, 1.

Mandel, P. and Edel-Harth, S. (1966). J. Neurochem. 13, 591.

Morest, D.K. (1969). Z. Anat. Entwickl.-Gesch. 128, 290.

Murthy, M.R.V. and Rappoport, D.A. (1964). Biochim. Biophys. Acta 95, 121.

Noback, C.R. and Purpura, D.P. (1961). J. Comp. Neurol. 117, 291.

Oja, S.S. (1966). Ann. Acad. Sci. Fennicae 125, 1.

Oja, S.S. (1972). J. Neurochem. 19, 2057.

Pasquini, J.M., Kaplún, B., Garcia, C.A. and Gomez, C.J. (1967). Brain Res. 6, 621.

Pysh, J.J. (1970). Brain Res. 18, 325.

Riege, W.H. (1971). Develop. Psychobiol. 4, 157.

Ringborn, U. (1966). Brain Res. 2, 296.

Rugh, R. (1968). Atompraxis 14, 1.

Schadé, J.P. and Baxter, C.F. (1960). Exp. Neurol. 2, 158.

Schadé, J.P. and Van Groeningen, W.B. (1961). Acta Anat. 47, 74.

Schadé, J.P. and Meeter, K. (1963). In "The Rhinencephalon and Related Structures" (W. Bargman and J.P. Schadé, eds.), Prog. Brain Res. 3, 89, Elsevier, Amsterdam.

Schadé, J.P., Meeter, K. and Van Groeningen, W.B. (1962). Acta Morphol. Neerl.-Scand. 5, 37.

Schjeide, O.A., I-San Lin, R. and de Vellis, J. (1968). Radiation Res. 33, 107.

Schonbach, J., Hu, K.H. and Friede, R. (1968). J. Comp. Neurol. 134, 21.

Smart, J.L. and Dobbing, J. (1971a). Brain Res. 28, 85.

Smart, J.L. and Dobbing, J. (1971b). Brain Res. 33, 303.

Sokoloff, L. and Roberts, P. (1971). In "Influence of Hormones on the Nervous System" (D.H. Ford, ed.), pp. 211-230, Karger AG, Basel.

Soriero, O. and Ford, D.H. (1971). In "Influence of Hormones on the Nervous System" (D.H. Ford, ed.), pp. 322-333, Karger AG, Basel.

Soriero, O. and Ford, D.H. (1973). In "The Neurobiology of Maturation and Aging" (D.H.Ford, ed.), Elsevier, Amsterdam (in press).

Tata, J.R. (1964). In "The Thyroid Gland" (R. Pitt-Rivers and W.R. Trotter, eds.), Vol. 1, Butterworths, London.

Vaccari, A., Maura, M., Marchi, M. and Cugurra, F. (1972). J. Neurochem. 19, 2453.

Vahvelainen, M. L. and Oja, S.S. (1969). Brain Res. 13,227.

Valcana, T., Hudson, D. and Timiras, P.S. (1972). J. Neurochem. 19, 2229.

Vernadakis, A. and Timiras, P.S. (1963). Am. J. Physiol. 205, 177.

Vernadakis, A. and Woodbury, D.M. (1962). Am. J. Physiol. 203, 748.

Vernadakis, A., Casper, R. and Timiras, P.S. (1968). Experientia 24, 237.

Yamagami, S., Fritz, R.R. and Rappoport, D.A. (1966). Biochim. Biophys. Acta 129, 532.

Zomzely, C.E., Roberts, S., Gruber, C.P. and Brown, D.M. (1968). J. Biol. Chem. 243, 5396.

TABLE 1

Apparent Michaelis Constants (K_m) and maximal velocities for incorporation (V_{max}) for tyrosine, phenylalanine and tryptophan into rat brain homogenates.

Age in Days	Tyrosine (5) K_m (μM)	Tyrosine (5) V_{max} (nMole/min/gm)	Phenylalanine (5) K_m (μM)	Phenylalanine (5) V_{max} (nMole/min/gm)	Tryptophan (4) K_m (μM)	Tryptophan (4) V_{max} (nMole/min/gm
1	34 ± 7	17.2 ± 1.6	71 ± 13	11.1 ± 1.0	481 ± 56	11.5 ± 1.0
7	41 ± 6	16.3 ± 1.0	79 ± 18	8.3 ± 2.1	487 ± 28	12.5 ± 0.4
21	53 ± 7	7.3 ± 1.2	201 ± 24	5.2 ± 0.7	641 ± 178	8.6 ± 1.8
60	126 ± 19	5.5 ± 1.4	287 ± 30	4.0 ± 0.4	865 ± 101	10.0 ± 1.1

The numbers in parenthesis indicate the number of experiments.
Adapted from Oja, _J. Neurochem._, _19_:2057-2069, 1972.

TABLE 2

Accumulation of ^{3}H-lysine into brain grey matter and neurons in relation to the volume of grey matter occupied by neurons and by the size of the neurons in the rat spinal cord.

Age in weeks	Percent grey matter occupied by neuronal soma[1]	nMoles ^{3}H-lysine accumulated per gram of grey matter	Weight ventral horn motoneurons in ngrams[2]	nMoles ^{3}H-lysine accumulated per gm ventral horn motoneurons
1	20.36	1.430	11.2	98.2
2	14.18	1.205	15.6	44.1
3	17.89	1.117	18.2	43.0
4	8.28	0.614	20.0	15.8
5	6.53	-	23.5	-
6	8.93	0.657	25.0	16.9
7	10.96	-	-	-
14	7.70	0.003	54.0	0.358

[1] Ford and Rhines, Acta Neurol. Scandinav. 45:529-539, 1969.
[2] Ford and Cohan, Acta Anat. 71:311-319, 1968.

Table 3

A comparison of the percent of the radioactivity present as I^{131}-triiodothyronine or its metabolites in rat brain at varying time intervals after intravenous injection of the labeled hormone as related to age.

Age	Time (Hours)	$T_3(+T_4)$ $^{131}I^{o}$ Mean	SE(±)*	MIT + DIT ^{131}I Mean	SE(±)	Iodide^{131} Mean	SE(±)
One Week	1/2	60.86	(3.81)	32.60	(1.42)	6.52	(0.98)
	1	49.99	(3.62)	28.57	(0.92)	21.43	(1.28)
	2	55.55	(7.22)	33.33	(1.64)	11.11	(1.72)
	4	55.85	(1.68)	29.45	(0.73)	14.81	(0.21)
	7	55.31	(2.17)	42.53	(0.96)	2.16	(0.41)
Two Weeks	1/2	64.90	(1.49)	23.40	(1.04)	11.70	(0.35)
	1	52.50	(3.26)	35.59	(0.47)	11.91	(1.09)
	2	69.45	(2.87)	20.43	(0.87)	10.11	(0.63)
	4	59.38	(1.49)	39.41	(0.93)	1.21	(0.19)
	7	72.73	(3.67)	9.30	(0.72)	17.97	(0.84)
Three Weeks	1/2	58.60	(2.82)	26.23	(1.17)	15.16	(0.68)
	1	79.96	(4.16)	17.30	(0.63)	3.74	(0.91)
	2	83.68	(5.28)	5.92	(0.31)	10.40	(0.47)
	4	59.61	(3.71)	30.78	(1.48)	9.62	(0.24)
	7	88.68	(3.29)	8.71	(0.99)	2.61	(0.09)
Four Weeks	1/2	78.31	(4.86)	9.41	(0.62)	12.28	(0.74)
	1	78.02	(4.77)	17.85	(1.48)	4.13	(0.19)
	2	72.08	(2.31)	24.86	(2.83)	3.08	(0.62)
	4	71.99	(2.16)	24.84	(3.89)	3.06	(0.47)
	7	81.39	(1.88)	17.38	(1.41)	1.33	(0.12)

*Represents the standard error of the mean (±).

^{o} ^{131}I-T_4 was present as a contaminant in small amounts in all the material obtained from Abbott Laboratories and never exceeded 2.5% of total amount of ^{131}I present. Traces of this ^{131}I-T_4 were found in most chromatograms. Cohan, et al., 1969.

Table 4

A comparison of the percent of the radioactivity present as I^{131}-triiodothyronine or its metabolites in the plasma of rats at varying time intervals after intravenous injection of the labeled hormone in relation to age.

Age	Time (Hours)	$T_3(+T_4)$ $^{131}I^{o}$ Mean	SE(±)*	MIT + DIT ^{131}I Mean	SE(±)	Iodide^{131} Mean	SE(±)
One Week	1/2	44.44	(3.77)	33.68	(1.96)	21.88	(1.46)
	1	22.90	(4.82)	24.80	(3.28)	42.20	(3.44)
	2	49.62	(3.14)	29.85	(1.33)	21.43	(2.62)
	4	20.80	(2.63)	41.62	(6.72)	37.58	(4.66)
	7	25.30	(3.85)	26.60	(5.24)	62.10	(5.97)
Two Weeks	1/2	52.99	(6.87)	17.70	(3.86)	29.31	(3.27)
	1	42.34	(4.72)	27.65	(5.99)	31.11	(4.16)
	2	30.79	(4.18)	25.51	(4.74)	43.70	(3.28)
	4	20.85	(0.92)	28.08	(2.31)	51.07	(3.79)
	7	28.21	(4.13)	38.62	(4.44)	33.07	(6.02)
Three Weeks	1/2	75.92	(2.67)	8.00	(0.20)	18.09	(4.16)
	1	55.46	(4.11)	19.12	(3.00)	26.42	(2.83)
	2	44.24	(4.69)	21.13	(3.31)	34.63	(2.16)
	4	38.50	(5.18)	23.00	(1.06)	38.50	(1.67)
	7	17.29	(5.10)	23.20	(4.03)	59.51	(3.21)
Four Weeks	1/2	71.52	(11.28)	12.01	(1.66)	16.46	(1.41)
	1	63.92	(4.73)	18.83	(1.51)	17.76	(1.38)
	2	47.12	(6.11)	13.76	(2.62)	39.11	(2.11)
	4	18.47	(2.38)	14.02	(3.29)	67.51	(4.89)
	7	11.96	(3.54)	19.18	(1.25)	69.12	(5.18)

Each value represents the mean of three animals.
*Represents the standard error of the mean (±).
o ^{131}I-T_4 was present as a contaminant in small amounts in all the materials obtained from Abbott Laboratories and never exceeded 2.5% of total amount of ^{131}I present. Traces of this ^{131}I-T_4 were found in most chromatograms.
Cohan, *et al.*, 1969.

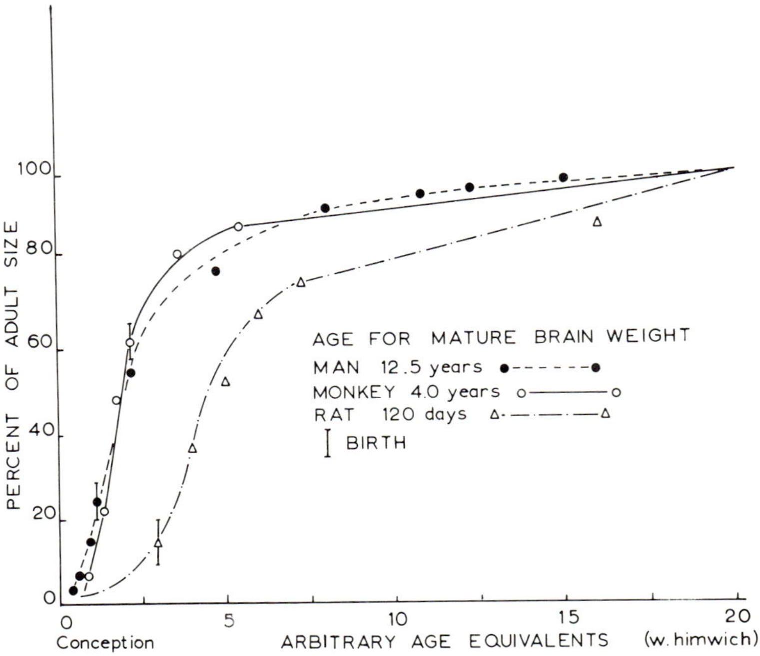

Fig. 1 A comparison of the relative growth rates of rat, monkey and human brains from near the time of conception until maximal growth is achieved. The weights are plotted in relation to percent of adult weight against arbitrary age units wherein the time from first development until maturity is broken up into 20 equal units and the size plotted accordingly. (From Himwich, W.A., <u>In</u> "The Neurobiology of Maturation and Aging", D.H. Ford, Ed., Elsevier, Amsterdam, in press.)

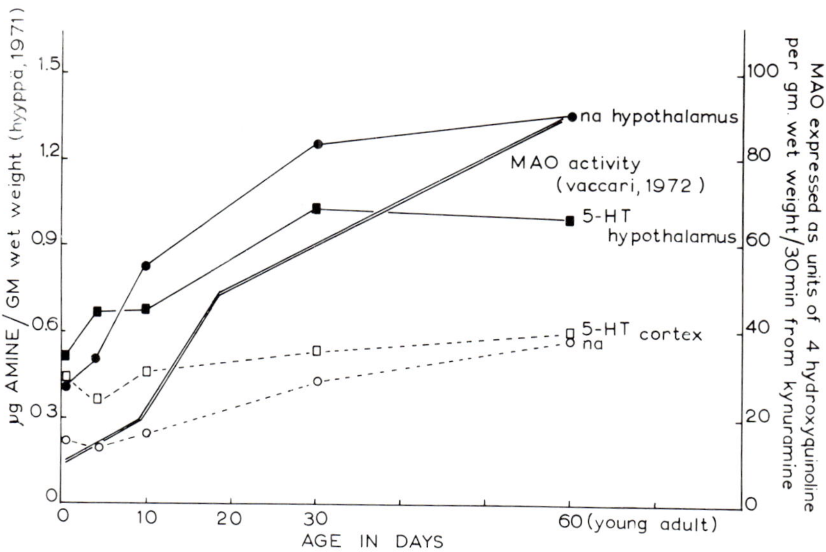

Fig. 2 A comparison of the levels of norepinephrine (NA) and serotonin (5-HT) in the hypothalamus and cerebral cortex of rats at different ages as related to the levels of monoamine oxidase activity (MAO). (From Vaccari, A., _et al_., 1972, _J_. _Neurochem_. _19_:2453-2457 and Hyyppä, M. 1971, _Experientia_ _27_:336-337.)

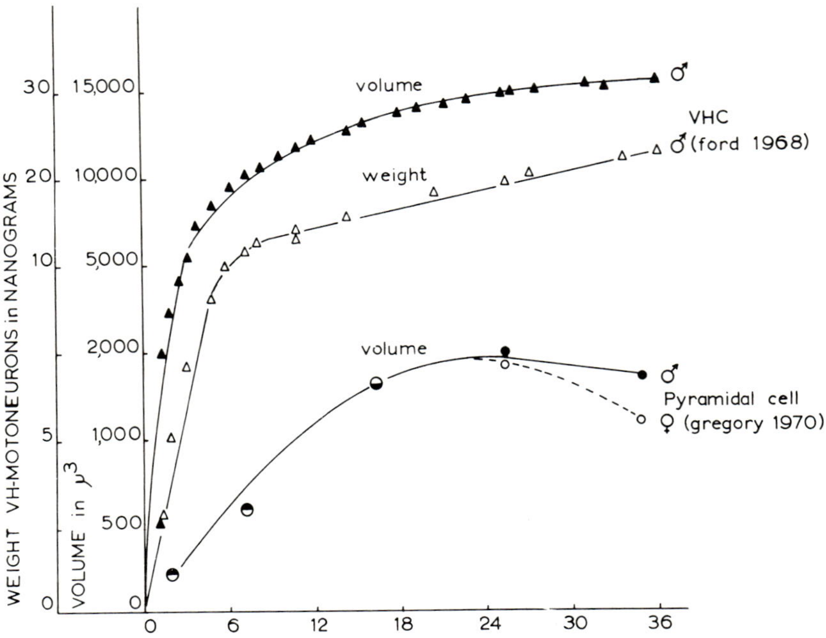

Fig. 3 A comparison of the growth of ventral horn motoneurons with that observed in pyramidal neurons of layer 5 of the cerebral cortex at the level of the anterior commissure (area 4 to 6) in relation to volume. The changes in the weights of ventral horn motoneurons with increasing age are also plotted. (From Ford, D.H. and Cohan, G. 1968, Acta Anat. 71:311-319 and Gregory, E. and Ford, D.H. 1970, Anat. Rec. 166:310.)

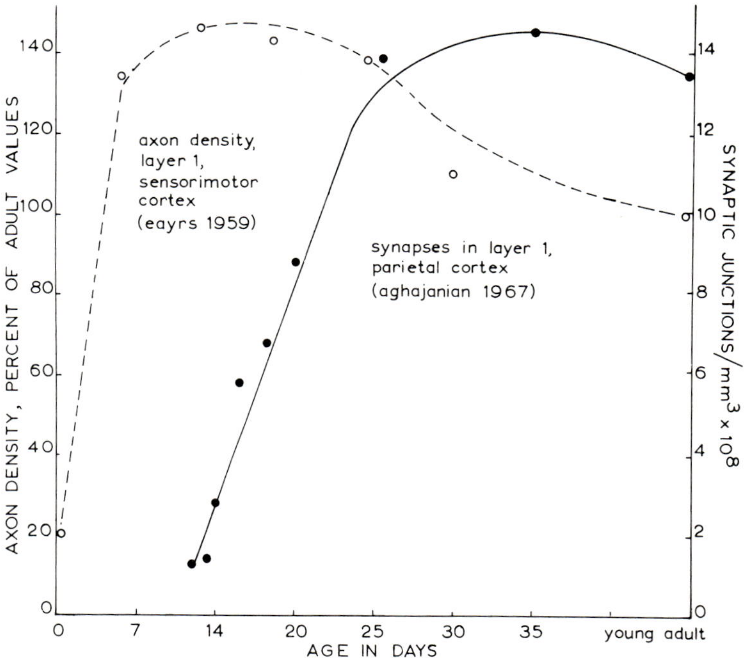

Fig. 4 A comparison of the increase in axon density with the increasing number of synaptic junctions observed in layer 1 of the cerebral cortex. (From Eayrs, J.T. and Goodhead, B. 1959, J. Anat. 93:385-402 and Aghajanian, G.K. and Bloom, F.E. 1967, Brain Res. 6:716-727.)

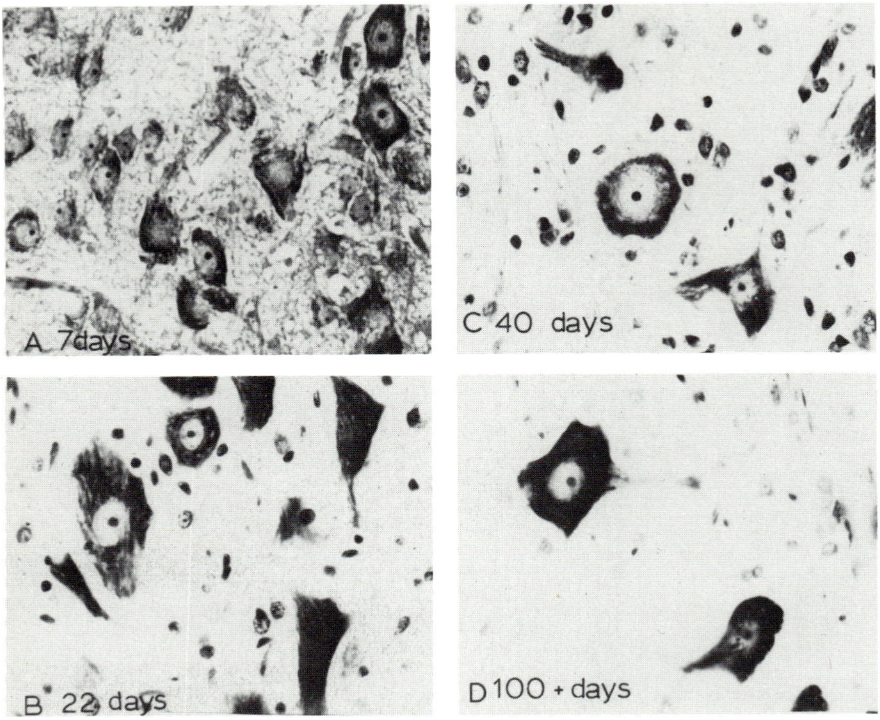

AGE (wks)	PERCENT VOLUME OCCUPIED BY NEURONS
1	20.36
2	14.18
3	17.89
4	8.28
5	6.53
6	8.93
7	10.96
14	7.70

Fig. 5 A photomicrographic demonstration of the change in volume of spinal cord grey matter occupied by neuronal soma during the maturational period. The magnification is the same for each age. Changes in the percent volume of grey matter occupied by neuronal soma are presented in tabular form. (From Ford, D.H. and Rhines, R. K. 1969, Acta Neurol. Scandinav. 45:41-52.)

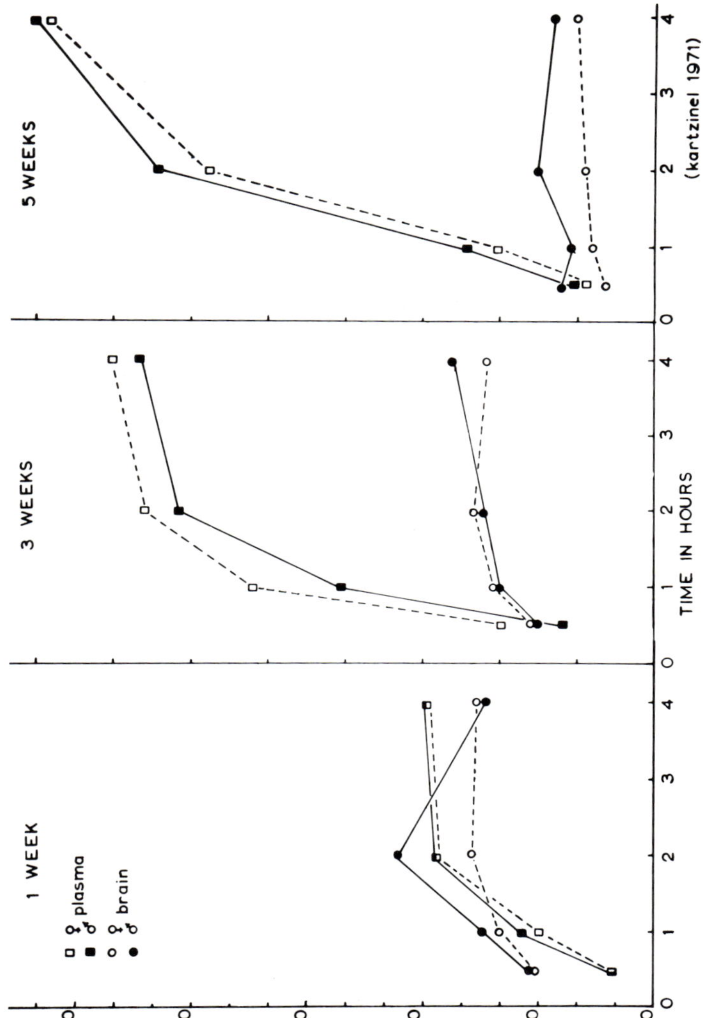

Fig. 6 A comparison of the amount of ^{3}H-lysine accumulated in brain and plasma proteins at 1, 3, and 5 weeks of age in male and female rats. (From Kartzinel, R., <u>et al</u>., 1971, <u>In</u> "Influence of Hormones on the Nervous System", D. H. Ford, Ed., S. Karger, Basel, pp. 296-305.)

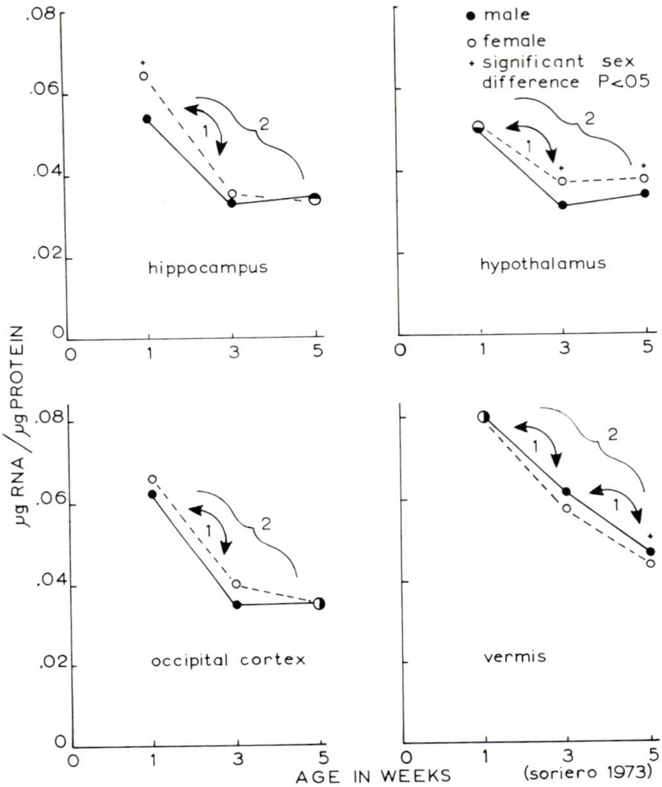

Fig. 7 A diagrammatic illustration of the changes in RNA/unit weight of protein in various brain areas in male and female rats at 1, 3, and 5 weeks of age. The + symbol indicates a significant sex difference ($P < 0.05$). The arched arrows signify a significant difference between 1 and 3 weeks or between 3 and 5 weeks. The inclusive symbol 2 indicates a significant difference between 1 and 5 weeks of age. (From Soriero, O. and Ford, D.H., 1971, In "Influence of Hormones on the Nervous System", D.H. Ford, Ed., S. Karger, Basel, pp. 322-333 and Soriero, O. and Ford, D.H. In "Neurobiology of Maturation and Aging", D.H. Ford, Ed., Elsevier, Amsterdam, in press.)

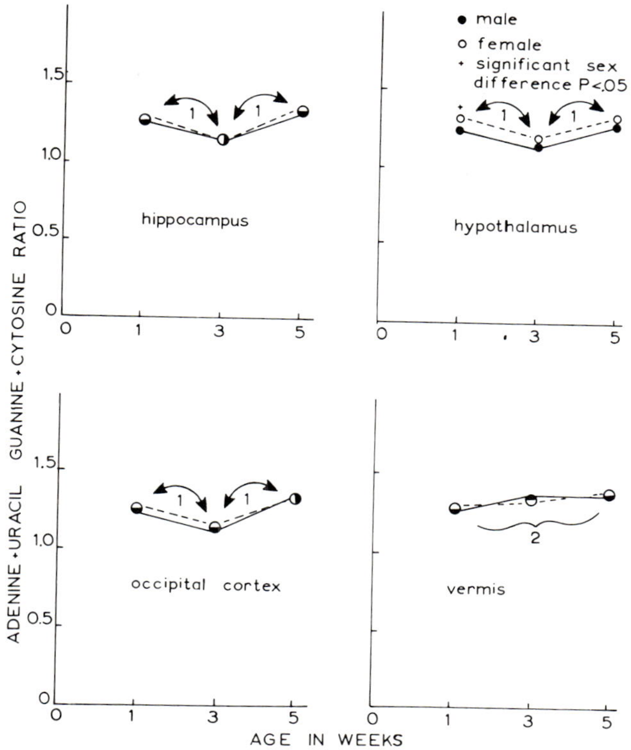

Fig. 8 A diagrammatic illustration of the changes in the adenine + uracil/guanine + cytosine ratio in various brain areas in male and female rats at 1, 3, and 5 weeks of age. The + symbol indicates a significant sex difference. The arched arrow 1 signifies a significant difference between 1 and 3 weeks and 3 and 5 weeks of age. The inclusive symbol 2 signifies a significant difference between 1 and 5 weeks of age. (From Soriero, O. and Ford, D.H., 1971, In "Influence of Hormones on the Nervous System", D. H. Ford, Ed., S. Karger, Basel, pp. 322-333 and Soriero, O. and Ford, D.H., In "Neurobiology of Maturation and Aging", D.H. Ford, Ed., Elsevier, Amsterdam, in press.)

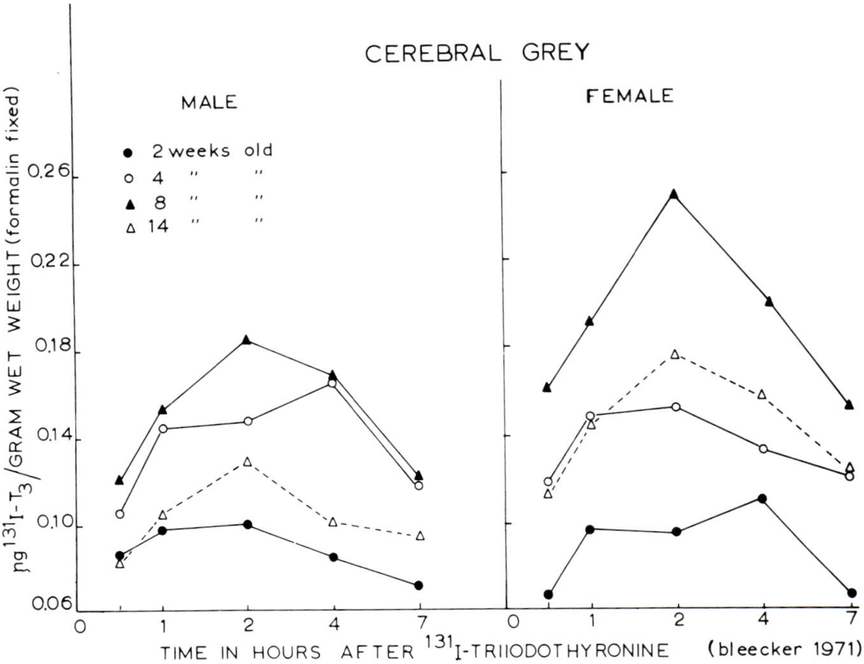

Fig. 9 A diagrammatic representation of the accumulation of ^{131}I-triiodothyronine in the cerebral cortex of male and female rats at 2, 4, 8, and 14 weeks of age. (From Bleecker, M.L., et al., 1971, In "Influence of Hormones on the Nervous System", D.H. Ford, Ed., Elsevier, Amsterdam, pp. 231-239.)

TROPHIC INFLUENCES IN THE MAMMALIAN CENTRAL NERVOUS SYSTEM

John C. Eccles

Departments of Physiology and Biophysics
State University of New York at Buffalo
School of Medicine
Buffalo, New York 14214

Introduction

Most investigators on the brain take the structure of the brain as given and proceed to study either this structure in itself or in one or another of its manifold performances. For example, it is now well established that the brain works as a neuronal machine, all information being coded in the impulse discharges of the individual cells. Thus very significant methods of investigation are concerned with studying these impulse discharges, which are essentially the "language" of communication in the brain. In the normal operation of the brain immensely complex patterns are "woven" in space and time by these impulse discharges. However, it is a serious omission to overlook a quite different system of communication between the neurones of the central nervous system, namely the so-called trophic communication. This system is still only vaguely understood; nevertheless its fundamental importance is undoubted. Consider for example the complex interacting sets of information that are responsible for the building of a brain with all its detailed connectivities established before usage. Consider again the factors concerned in the maintenance of the brain as a plastic structure capable of modification according to usage, which, of course, gives the brain its capacity to learn; that is to store information that can be retrieved. Finally, there are the factors concerned in regression and degeneration of neural structures and the limited regeneration that is possible even in the adult brain, although there is eventually a progressive failure in the aging process. Trophic influences may be defined as those factors concerned in the growth, maintenance and regression of nerve cells either as a whole or of an extrasomatic element, such as, for example, the dependence of the axon on trophic influences from the soma.

Neuromuscular Synapses

The development and aging process in neuromuscular synapses has been studied in normal mammals by Barker and Ip (1966). They described an endplate as undergoing an aging and degeneration and being replaced by a new endplate formed from a collateral sprout of the same motor axon. The continuous processes of endplate regression and regeneration in normal muscles have been reported by other investigators. However, according to Tuffery (1971), these are not linked processes, i.e., degeneration inducing regeneration. On the contrary, there is throughout life a continuous process of endplate elaboration. Eventually, even up to half of the motor axons branch proximal to their terminal arborization, endplates, in this way, being supplied by two or more myelinated fibers. Concurrently, there may be degeneration of endplates with no replacement. Thus, with aging there are fewer muscle fibers, such residual fibers being larger and supplied by more complex endplates.

Regression and Regeneration in Central Synapses

Sotelo and Palay (1971) have described concurrent processes of regression and regeneration of synapses in the adult mammalian central nervous system. So far these observations have been made in Deiters nucleus and in the gracilis nucleus of both rat and cat, in the cerebellar nuclei of the cat, and in the area postrema of the rat. It can be assumed that they are of quite general occurrence in the normal adult central nervous system. Degeneration of synaptic knobs is indicated by a remarkable series of structural changes, particularly in the organelles, there being a general resemblance to the changes observed in various degenerative diseases. Usually, in the electron microscopic pictures, only two or three of the structural changes are observed in any one synaptic knob, but some large swollen synaptic knobs provide a remarkable display of almost all of the ultrastructural features of degeneration: hyperplasia of cisternal profiles; concentric laminar arrays; assemblies of closely packed tubules; abnormal mitochondria; increase in the size and density of lysosomes; and depletion of synaptic vesicles. There may be only a few vesicles in proximity with the dense membrane profiles of a synaptic site. In a few cases, a synaptic knob of normal structure can be seen budding off from a large degenerating terminal. Sotelo and Palay (1971) postulate that this linked degeneration and regeneration gives a continuous remodelling of the axonal terminals that occurs with different rates according to the animal species and the location within the brain. They further postulate that, if this plasticity extends to dendrites as well as to axonal terminals, the synaptic plasticity provides a structural basis for the growth theory of learning. This remarkable evidence for regression and regeneration of synapses reveals that the adult mammalian nervous system is more plastic than had been generally assumed. In this light, we will now reconsider some of the classical experimental attempts to reveal plasticity by testing for compensatory responses to operative procedures.

Investigations on Plastic Reactions of the Spinal Cord

Remarkable investigations were carried out by Weiss and Sperry on larval amphibians, in which functional recovery of specific reactions occurred following transplantation of limbs and receptor organs and the cross-union of nerve trunks. Sperry (1945) interpreted these findings as showing that the reconstitution occurred because the nerve fibers of the severed pathways were guided by specific chemical specificities to make synapses on "appropriate" neuronal targets. However, he failed to discover any signs of functional recovery as tested by reflex responses when nerves of mammalian limbs were cross-unioned even in very young animals. In 1945 Sperry reviewed all of the experimental evidence for plastic changes in the mammalian central nervous system, and concluded that no such changes had been demonstrated. Nevertheless, it must be assumed that in fetal life the complex and specific neuronal connectivities must be established by processes of chemical sensing comparable with those demonstrated in larval amphibians.

Early in the 1960s we (reviewed in Eccles, 1963)

reinvestigated the effects of nerve crossing in the mammalian spinal cord because it was then possible to make a more refined study than in the much earlier experiments of Sperry. The nerve cross-unions were made in very young kittens (10 to 28 days old) and 6 to 17 months later the sensitive and discriminative technique of intracellular recording was employed in order to detect even slight remodellings of the monosynaptic pathways from the annulospiral endings of muscle via the group Ia afferent fibers. This specific testing procedure was used because advantage could be taken of the precise patterns of monosynaptic excitation that had been established in investigations on over 2000 motoneurones. It had thus been shown that monosynaptic excitation was almost exclusively exerted by group Ia fibers on motoneurones of that muscle or of a synergic muscle. Deviations from this rule were rare and always very weak.

There are two aspects of the hypothesis that specific chemical sensing guides functional remodelling of central connections following nerve cross-union. In the first place, it is assumed that muscles can trophically influence the motoneurones innervating them. One aspect of the hypothesis relates to the growth of Ia monosynaptic connections to motoneurones, which are in accord with their newly acquired functions resulting from the nerve cross-union. It may be called "growth specificity". The other aspect is concerned with the regression of the monosynaptic connections which are rendered inappropriate by the changed motoneuronal function resulting from the nerve cross-union. It may be called "regression-specificity". These processes are not mutually exclusive. They are, in fact, two aspects of the hypothesis of myotypic specification formulated by Weiss and Sperry. Both processes may cooperate in the reestablishment of appropriate patterns of connection after the nerve cross-union.

Fig. 1A shows diagrammatically the normal monosynaptic connectivities between two pairs of synergic muscles. The hundreds of Ia afferent fibers and motoneurones for each muscle are represented singly. In all cases, the homonymous innervation is shown by the larger synaptic knob. Insofar as monosynaptic innervation is concerned, there is no connection normally between the two pairs of synergists, which are chosen for the operative cross-union because of this characteristic. The cross-union is shown in Fig. 1B.

The operation had been performed on kittens a few days old and many months had been allowed for recovery of the peripheral connections by nerve regeneration. In the testing experiments, nerve stimulation was applied to the nerves proximal to the cross-union, as indicated, and the monosynaptic responses of motoneurones were observed by intracellular recording. In a number of kittens of the same age, control experiments testing for the effect of nerve section alone were performed by the operation of section and self-union. These control experiments are important because sectioning of the muscle nerves in young kittens results in the chromatolytic death of about two thirds of both afferent and efferent fibers to a muscle, and this alone might induce changes in central connectivities.

In the final analysis of the results it was shown that with some species of cross-union there was a small, but statistically significant development of monosynaptic excitatory synapses from the afferent fibers of an intact pathway (SA_2 of Fig. 1B) to motoneurones that had acquired synergism because of the cross-union -- the broken line of Fig. 1B. This is an example of the postulated "growth-specificity". The postulated "regression-specificity" was also observed as a statistically significant reduction of the monosynaptic excitation exerted by the Ia fibers of the cross-unioned muscle to motoneurones of its erstwhile synergist. This reduction is indicated by the wavy line over the pathway from A_1 to SMN_1. This regression was of course tested against the self-unioned controls so as to eliminate the complications of chromatolytic death of about two-thirds of the severed Ia afferent fibers.

In evaluating the significance of these demonstrations that myotypic specification remodels central connections in young mammals, it must be recognized that the observed effects, though statistically significant in our samples of many hundreds of motoneurones show that only small changes were effected. In part, these changes have functional meaning, but in the experimental series there were statistically significant cases of central remodelling that apparently had no functional meaning and hence are unrelated to the present form of the myotypic specification hypothesis. In fact, it was suggested that the remodelling may be an aftermath of the chromatolytic damage suffered by both the Ia afferent neurones and the motoneurones. Many die and those that recover may have been through a phase of increased plasticity.

In conclusion, it can be stated that, although the mammalian spinal cord offers the advantage of precise study, it may be unsuitable because its plasticity is at such a low level even very early in postnatal life. It is therefore of great interest that at higher levels of the mammalian central nervous system there are now several investigations revealing that operative lesions may lead to plastic reconstructions.

Modification of Synaptic Connectivities by Operative Procedures at Higher Levels of the Central Nervous System

Recent experimental studies at the higher levels of the mammalian central nervous system have been concerned with axonal growths subsequent to surgically produced degenerations. The most favorable conditions are provided when the degenerating axonal terminals and synapses are interspersed with normal fibers that are synapsing on the same neurones.

As illustrated in Fig. 2, the septal nuclei provide ideal conditions for the experimental investigations of Raisman (1969). The two principal inputs to these nuclei are the fimbrial pathway from the hippocampus and the medial forebrain bundle (MFB) from the hypothalamus. The former input forms synapses almost exclusively on the dendrites of septal cells, while the latter input ends on both dendrites and somata (Fig. 2A). After sectioning of either pathway in adult rats (3-6 months old) there was convincing evidence that the fibers of the other pathway sprouted (cf. Fig. 2B,C) to occupy the vacated synaptic sites. For example, some weeks later, EM studies showed that the fimbrial fibers now innervated a considerable number of synapses on the somata (Fig. 2C), and the terminals of the MFB fibers made many double synaptic sites as indicated in Fig. 2B. It appears that there has been a loss of the embryonic growth specificity, so that collaterals growing from the intact axons now heterotypically innervate synaptic sites originally reserved for and occupied by the other input. Raisman (1969) regards this heterotypic growth of synapses as being functionally meaningless. Nevertheless, this regeneration is of great interest because it shows that axonal sprouting and synaptic formation can occur in the adult rat, but only at micro-distances. Raisman further suggests that this regeneration may be aided by the chromatolytic reaction of the septal neurones in the same manner as has been suggested for motoneurones. Since the axons of the septal neurones are in both the fimbria and the MFB, they were sectioned in the initial operation. Possibly the glial cells also aid in this heterotypic regeneration in the same manner as the Schwann cells in the case of peripheral regeneration. Two important negative findings are that the sectioned fibers make only abortive growths and do not regenerate over the distances of millimeters along their degenerating pathways and that there is no evidence for development of new synaptic sites on the septal cells, there being merely heterotypic reinnervation of old sites.

Lund and Lund (1971) have also provided evidence of heterotypic synaptic regeneration in the superior colliculus of both young and adult rats after removal of one eye. Some 4-5 months post-operatively, there was found to be an excess of synapses with flattened vesicles and symmetric contacts. They therefore suggest that the terminal fibers of other inputs to the superior colliculus sprout collaterals that occupy the synaptic sites vacated by the degenerated optic fibers. This evidence is less convincing than the changes seen by Raisman in the septal nuclei, but it is in good accord with the evidence.

It would be expected that more favorable conditions for synaptic regeneration would occur in very young animals when the normal developmental processes are still acting. That this indeed seems to be the case is shown by two investigations in young cats (7-9 days postnatal) and rats (10-11 days postnatal).

When the eye of an adult cat or of a kitten 20 days old was removed, Guillery (1972) found that 4 months to 4 years later there was no compensatory growth into the denervated laminae of the lateral geniculate body from the adjacent innervated laminae. This failure was disclosed by the lack of any degenerating fibers in the originally denervated laminae 4 to 13 days after removal of the second eye. In contrast, when the first operation was performed on kittens 7 to 9 days old, there were, after the second operation, degenerating fibers in the denervated laminae. This reinnervated zone was close to the normally innervated laminae, as illustrated in Fig. 3; hence Guillery suggested that probably the normally growing fibers in the young animal continued on into the denervated laminae and that strictly speaking there was no new sprouting of axon collaterals. At least to some extent the innervation of the denervated laminae is functional, since it contributes to the maintenance of the border cells.

Wall and Egger (1971) have reported a similar limited regeneration in marginal zones of a denervated thalamic region. Likewise, they attribute this response to a continued axonal growth into the denervated zone.

A very significant study has recently been made by Steward, *et al.*(1973) on the innervation pathways from the entorhinal cortex to the hippocampus. By degeneration techniques (Fig. 4A) it has been demonstrated that the entorhinal cortex of the one side ipsilaterally innervates the distal two-thirds of the dendrites of the granule cells and the distal dendrites of the pyramidal cells of the CA_3 region of the hippocampus. In addition, there is a small distribution to the apical dendrites of the pyramidal cells of the CA_1 region of both sides. However, there is no innervation of the contralateral granule cells (Fig. 4A, B). When the entorhinal cortex of one side is ablated in rats 10-11 days old, degeneration experiments some weeks later show that the contralateral entorhinal cortex has established fiber growth and synapses on the granule cell dendrites. This is shown by the distribution of degenerating fibers when that cortex is later excised, as shown in Fig. 4C,D. This growth of crossed temperodentate fibers appears to reoccupy the synaptic territory vacated by the degenerated ipsilateral entorhinal fibers. Presumably this growth occurs from the entorhinal fibers giving the crossed innervation of those CA_1 pyramidal cells that are in close proximity to the dentate granule cells. Nevertheless, the fiber growth would have to occur across the hippocampal fissure and a distance of several hundred microns would have to be travelled to give the sparse reinnervation of the ventral leaf of the dentate gyrus that is shown in Fig. 4D. The authors point out that, at the time of the initial operation, the innervation of the hippocampus from the entorhinal cortex was at a very early stage, only 5% of the mature terminals being formed; hence the regenerative response could be accomplished merely be a continuous growth of actively growing fibers in the manner suggested for the lateral geniculate (cf. Fig. 3).

The most interesting finding by Steward, *et al.* (1973)

is that the synapses formed by the crossed temperodentate fibers are functionally effective. As would be expected from the fiber distribution shown in Fig. 4A, stimulation of the contralateral entorhinal cortex does not normally evoke any short latency excitation of the dentate granule cells. In contrast, 25 days after excision of the ipsilateral entorhinal cortex there was quite a large crossed excitation. Stimulation of the entorhinal cortex evoked a field potential signalling that there was monosynaptic excitation of the granule cell dendrites at the reinnervated synaptic sites (cf. Fig. 4C,D). This excitation was even powerful enough to evoke impulse discharges from the granule cells. This is the first demonstration that these heterotypic synaptic regenerations are functionally effective; but they may not be functionally meaningful. It is not yet known if there is any fiber growth and reinnervation after entorhinal ablation in the adult.

Summary

In summary, it can be stated that at higher levels of the central nervous system in young mammals degeneration of fibers with their synapses results in a remarkable growth of adjacent intact fibers so that there is reoccupation of vacated synaptic sites. It can be postulated that the trophic signal is provided, in part at least, by the degenerating fibers, in the manner that has been well established in the peripheral nervous system. This trophic influence may be mediated by glial cells, just as occurs with Schwann cells in the peripheral nervous system. Doubtless the vacated synaptic sites also contribute attractive influences, so ensuring their reoccupation, even if it be by synaptic terminals which, in the original growth, avoided these sites because of their different specificities. These regenerations in young animals occur only for short distances -- a few hundred microns at the most. In adult mammals, regeneration has been observed only in special situations where the new growths would be for tens of microns at the most. After cross-union experiments on the spinal cords of young mammals, growth giving reconstitution of synapses is quite unusual, but it <u>has</u> been demonstrated. We can conclude that, contrary to the generally accepted belief, there is a limited amount of regeneration at the higher levels of the mammalian nervous system. It is but a fragile remainder of the organized growth patterns of fetal life, that must have been operating at subtle levels of specificity in order to build the nervous system with the fully fashioned connections that are established before its first activities.

The regenerations illustrated in Figs. 2-4 result in synaptic connections different from those normally existing, i.e. they are heterotypic. It would be difficult technically to show that homotypic regenerations also occur for distances of a few tens of microns, which seems to be the utmost range for heterotypic regeneration in all cases but the ventral leaflet of the fascia dentata in Fig. 4D. In the experiments carried out so far, a catastrophic lesion is produced causing degeneration of all fibers of a particular type. Homotypic regeneration is thus excluded. Nevertheless, the observed heterotypic regenerations strongly support the hypothesis that homotypic regenerations do occur. Because the embryonically operating specificities probably still operate, it would be expected that homotypic regenerations would be in excess of the observed heterotypic. Since short range regenerations occur in the adult central nervous system (cf. Fig. 2) in order to occupy vacated synaptic sites, it can be postulated that degenerations of individual neurones in the aging brain may be in part compensated for by homotypic regeneration. One can envisage that the vacated synaptic sites are occupied by sprouting from adjacent presynaptic fibers giving a largely homotypic reoccupation.

Thus, there would be two processes of compensation for the degenerations of the aging process. In one, there is a coupled synaptic degeneration and regeneration that has been demonstrated by Sotelo and Palay (1971). In the other, individual neuronal death is compensated at least in part by homotypic reoccupation of the vacated synaptic sites. Since there is great redundancy in the neuronal composition of central pathways, no serious deficiencies in performance would be expected to arise when there is this compensatory reoccupation of synaptic sites. The normal complement of synaptic power on neurones may decline but little, giving normal levels of neuronal performance. At the most there may be some loss of integrative subtlety because of the decline of the levels of divergence and of convergence in the neuronal connections. These conclusions obtain only for relatively mild and randomly dispersed neuronal degenerations, not for more severe degenerations having a concentrated distribution.

REFERENCES

Barker, D. and Ip, M.C. (1966). Proc. Royal Soc. B 163, 538.

Eccles, J.C. (1963). In "The Effect of Use and Disuse on Neuromuscular Functions." Czechoslovak Acad. Sci. Prague.

Guillery, R.W. (1972). J. Comp. Neurol. 146, 407.

Lund, R.D. and Lund, J.S. (1971). Science 171, 804.

Raisman, G. (1969). Brain Res. 14, 25.

Sotelo, C. and Palay, S.L. (1971). Lab Investigation 25, 653.

Sperry, R.W. (1945). Quart. Rev. Biol. 20, 311.

Steward, O., Cotman, C.W. and Lynch, G.S. (1973). Exp. Brain Res. (In press).

Tuffery, A.R. (1971). J. Anat. 110, 221.

Wall, P.D. and Egger, M.D. (1971). Nature 232, 542.

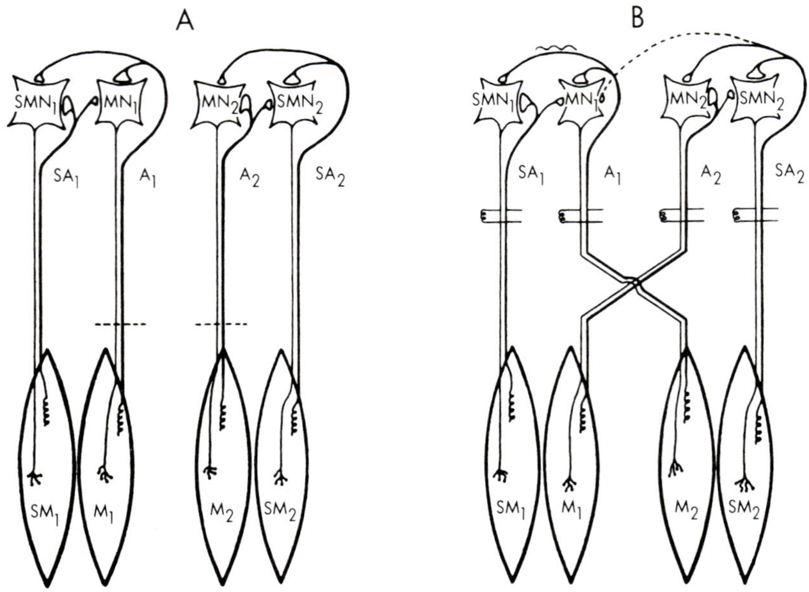

Fig. 1 A: Diagrammatic representation of monosynaptic pathways for two pairs of synergic muscles: M_1 and SM_1, M_2 and SM_2. The afferent fibers, A_1, SA_1, A_2, SA_2, respectively, from the annulospiral endings are seen to make monosynaptic connections to motoneurones of their own muscle (homonymous endings) and of the synergic muscle (heteronymous endings). The larger synaptic knobs for the homonymous endings symbolize the more powerful excitatory action. The broken lines drawn across the nerves to M_1 and M_2 muscles indicate the site of section and self-union in the control experiments. B: Diagrammatic representation of cross-union of the nerves to M_1 and M_2 muscles with regeneration such as occurred for the three types of cross-union per X MG, LGS X Pl and DP X MG described (Eccles, 1963). Broken line from SA_2 to MN_1 represents the new connections which appear to occur under certain conditions (see text), and which would be due to growth-specificity. The wavy line above the connection from A_1 to SMN_1 symbolizes the decreased synaptic excitatory action which appears to occur under certain conditions (see text), and which would be due to regression-specificity. Stimulating electrodes are shown in B. (Eccles, 1963).

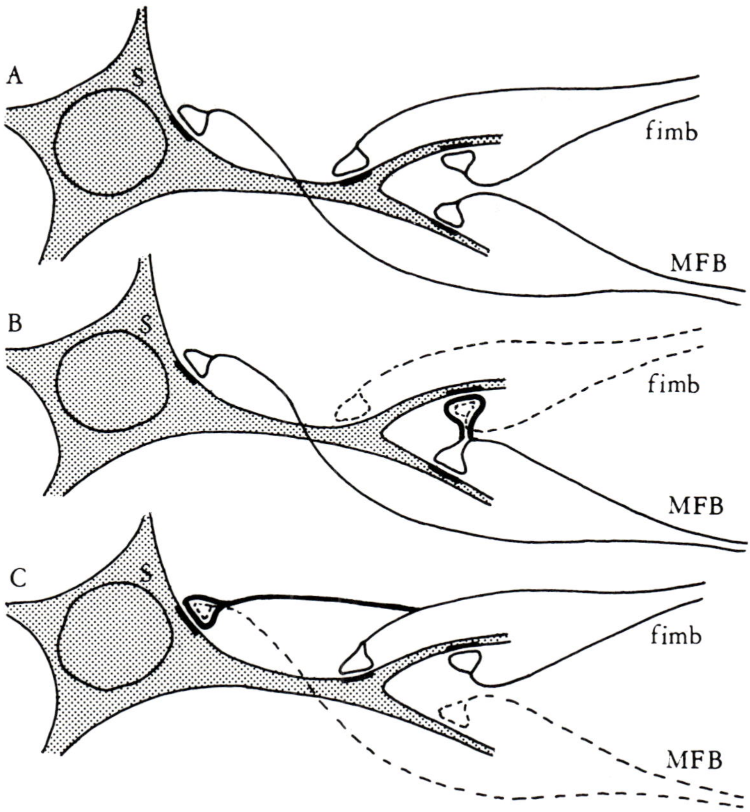

Fig. 2 Schematic representation of synaptic connections to septal cells. A: In the normal situation, afferents from the medial forebrain bundle (MFB) terminate in boutons on the cell soma (S) and on dendrites, while the fimbrial fibers (fimb) are restricted in termination to the dendrites. B: Several weeks after a lesion of the fimbria, the medial forebrain bundle terminals extend across from their own sites to occupy the vacated sites, thus forming double synapses. (Degenerated connections: discontinuous line; presumed plastic changes: heavy black line.) C: Several weeks after a lesion of the medial forebrain bundle, the fimbrial fibers now give rise to terminals occupying somatic sites, which are presumably those vacated as a result of the former lesion. (Raisman, 1969.)

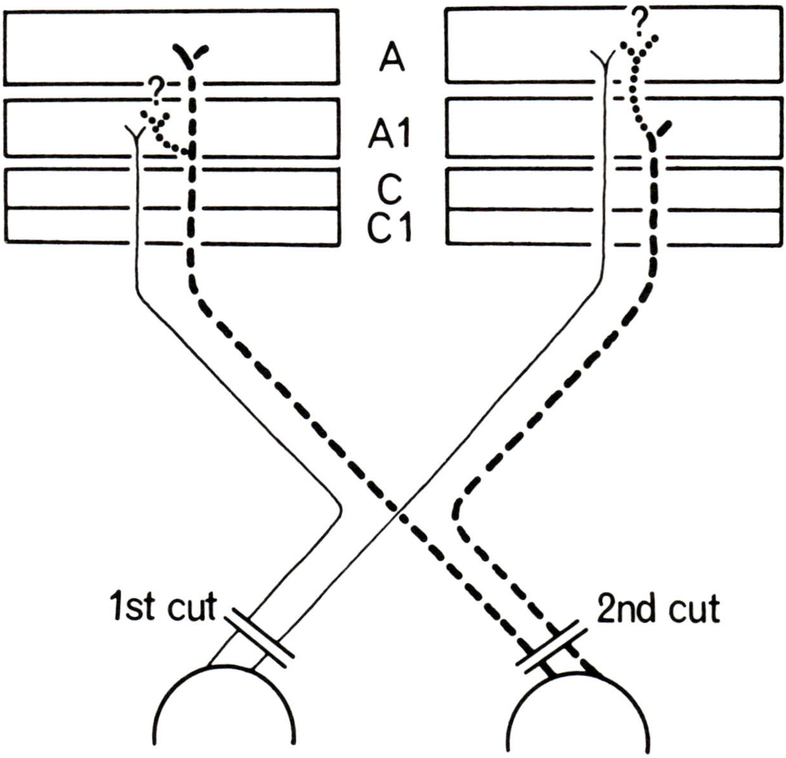

Fig. 3 Schema to show the design of the experiments. The first cut produced degeneration in the left retinofugal axons, which are shown as thin continuous lines. After a period of time sufficient for complete removal of the debris, the second cut produced degeneration in the right retinofugal axons, which are shown as thick interrupted lines, and which were stained by the Nauta method. If collateral sprouting occurred after the first operation, then the axons from the right eye will have sent branches into regions that were initially innervated by the left eye, as indicated by the dotted lines, and these sprouts will also have degenerated after the second operation. Laminae A, A1, C and C1 are shown, but the optic nerve terminals and presumed sprouts are shown for the A laminae only. (Guillery, 1972.)

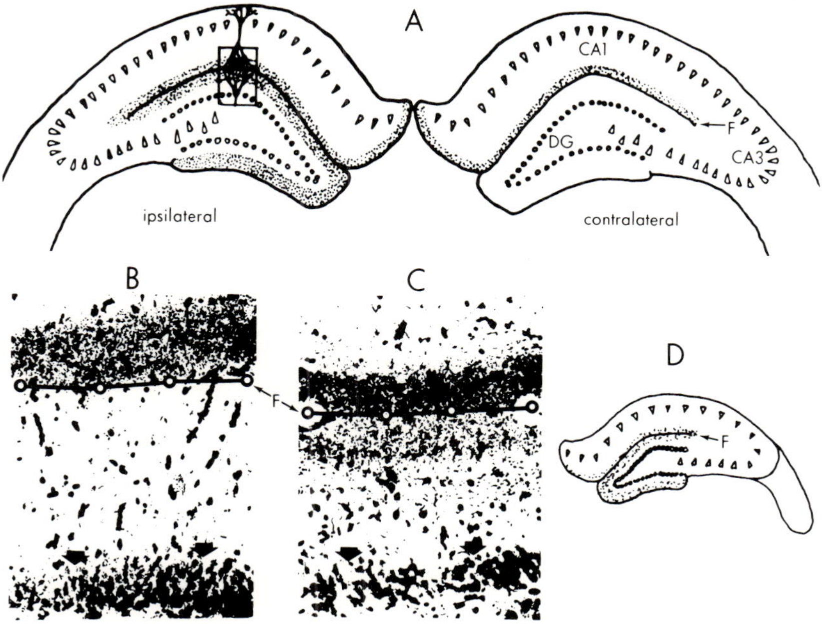

Fig. 4 Projections of the entorhinal cortex to the hippocampus and dentate gyrus. A: A schematic representation of the hippocampal formation in coronal section indicates the cellular divisions of the hippocampus (CA1 and CA3) and the dentate gyrus (DG). The orientation of a granule cell of the dorsal leaf, and a pyramidal cell of the CA1 hippocampus is indicated on the left. The terminal field of the normal entorhinal projection is indicated by the dots. B,C: The distribution of contralateral entorhinal afferents to the hippocampal formation is traced with the Fink-Heimer (1967) method. B shows the distribution of contralateral entorhinal afferents in the normal animal, the degeneration being restricted to the CA1. The line through the open circles is the hippocampal fissure (F). C shows a similar location in an experimental animal when ipsilateral entorhinal afferents had been removed at 10 days of age. The normal site of termination is evident above the hippocampal fissure, but in addition, there is a new projection which invades the molecular layer of the dentate gyrus immediately below the hippocampal fissure. D shows in a section similar to that of A (contralateral) the distribution of the degeneration seen in a small section (C). It shows that the contralateral entorhinal projection now has spread below the hippocampal fissure (F) and even round to the ventral leaf of the dentate gyrus.

GENESIS OF NEURONAL LOCUS SPECIFICITY

Marcus Jacobson*

Department of Biophysics
The Johns Hopkins University
Baltimore, Maryland 21218

The location of nerve cells and the trajectories of nerve fibers are remarkably similar in all individuals of the same species. Many observations over the past century have confirmed this invariance of neural circuitry in many different species of animals and there are also many examples showing that the assembly of the components of the nervous system in the embryo proceeds along orderly, nonrandom lines. The observations led to the introduction of the term "neuronal specificity" about thirty years ago, to denote the singular features which distinguish one type of nerve cell from another. This term has been applied uncritically to at least two major differences between various types of neurons, based firstly upon the differences in their positions and secondly on their structural differences. Therefore, we ought to make a clear distinction between _neuronal phenotypic specificity_ when referring to the morphological differences between various types of nerve cells, and _neuronal locus specificity_ when referring to the unique and specific position-dependent properties that nerve cells exhibit.

Consider the example of the visual system in which neuronal phenotypic specificity is displayed by the various types of nerve cells that are found, for example, in the retina. Retinal ganglion cells differ in their morphology from retinal bipolar, amacrine, horizontal, or photoreceptor cells. Not only are cells of different types clearly found in different positions, but cells of the same

*Present Address: Department of Physiology and Biophysics, University of Miami School of Medicine, Miami, Florida 33152

neuronal phenotype may also be arrayed in a spatial pattern and have significant position-dependent differences. These position-dependent differences are well exhibited by the retinal ganglion cells, each of which sends its axon to a specific locus in the brain, so that their spatial order is projected as a retinotopic map into the visual centers of the brain. To identify this type of specificity clearly, we recently introduced the term "neuronal locus specificity" and defined it as the property of the individual retinal ganglion cell which predisposes its axon to terminate and synapse at a particular locus in the retinotectal map (Hunt and Jacobson, 1972a,b; 1973).

In normal frogs, ganglion cells at a particular retinal position always connect with a particular place in the optic tectum. Thus, the spatial pattern of individual retinal axon terminals in the tectum reduplicates the spatial relationship of the corresponding retinal ganglion cells. Thus, if a microelectrode is lowered into the tectum at a succession of positions further and further back on the tectum, one can record nerve action potentials in the electrode at each of these successive positions only by providing the frog with a visual stimulus at appropriate and more lateral positions in the visual field. In this manner one can map the retinotectal projection of the optic nerve terminals to the tectum. Such a map gives an indication of the position-dependent properties of the retinal ganglion cells which predispose each axon to terminate at a unique locus in the tectum. Because the map is obtained from presynaptic terminals, it does not show whether those terminals have formed functional synaptic connections in the tectum. There are means for recording postsynaptically in the tectum and for assaying the functional efficiency of the retinotectal connections, but in this paper we deal only with the loci of presynaptic terminals which serve as an assay of the position-dependent properties of the retinal cells. The retinotectal projection is used as a convenient assay of the locus specificities of the retinal ganglion cells, and not as an assay of functional connectivity between the eye and the brain.

In order to study the developmental origins of the position-dependent properties in the retinal ganglion cells our experimental strategy was to reposition one eye of the embryo of the clawed frog, <u>Xenopus laevis</u>, at various stages of development before the eye had started forming nervous connections with the brain. The eye was either inverted *in situ*, within the ocular orbit, or it was transplanted to another position on the body, or it was explanted into tissue culture for some time. In all cases the eye was then reintroduced to the orbit in order to assay the resulting retinotectal projection.

The first type of experiment was to excise the eye rudiment at various embryonic stages and then simply to reimplant it in different orientations in its own ocular orbit or, as shown in figure 1, transplant it from a donor to a carrier at the same stage of development (Jacobson, 1967; 1968). When the eye was rotated at embryonic stage 28 it gave rise to a normal retinotectal projection, when mapped after metamorphosis. However, when an eye rotation occurred a few hours later at embryonic stage 30 a retinotectal projection developed that was inverted in the anteroposterior axis of the retina, but normal in its dorsoventral axis. Slightly later, at stage 31, an eye rotation led to complete inversion of the retinotectal map. These experiments show that there is a change in the embryo, during a five to ten hour *critical period* between stages 28 to 32, during which there is a change in response of the retinotectal system to 180° rotation of the eye. The experiments permit three main conclusions:

First, the set of locus specificities that ultimately develop in an eye rotated before the critical period is spatially organized in accordance with the postoperative positions of the retinal cells and does not depend on the cells' preoperative positions.

On the other hand, in an eye rotated after the critical period, the set of locus specificities that ultimately develops is determined by the preoperative positions of the retinal cells and does not pay heed to their postoperative positions. By rotating an eye in the middle of the critical period, at about stage 30, the set of position-dependent properties that develops in the retina has an anteroposterior component which is appropriate to the eye's preoperative position but the dorsoventral component is appropriate to its postoperative position. Thus, the position-dependence of locus specificity has two axial components, one related to the ganglion cell's position in the anteroposterior axis of the retina and the other to the cell's position in the dorsoventral axis of the retina.

Finally, although the eye at stage 32 contains only a

few hundred retinal ganglion cells, and retinal axons have not yet grown out of the eye, rotation of the eye at stage 32 results in corresponding rotation of the entire retinotectal map of the adult eye which contains about 500,000 retinal ganglion cells. Apparently a developmental program has been established in the embryo that affects the entire set of specificities that will arise in the adult retina.

Two main limitations of such an experimental analysis should be emphasized here. The first relates to the long delay between the experimental manipulation of the embryonic eye rudiment and the final mapping of the ultimate set of locus specificities as they are expressed in the retinotectal map of the adult frog. During the intervening period there is a protracted process of generation of retinal and tectal cells, the growth of the retinal nerve fibers into the brain, and the formation of retinotectal connections. Although the experimental analysis shows that the complete set of locus specificities that finally develops in the adult retina is specified (or determined) during a short critical period in the embryo at stages 29 to 32, we cannot infer anything about the cellular mechanisms or the histogenetic programs that give rise to the spatial deployment of locus specificities and their expression during morphogenesis of the retinotectal map. Another limitation relates to the information that can be obtained from the map itself. The map provides no more than relative information about the disposition of the position-dependent properties across the retinal cell population. The map does not show which locus specificities are present; it only shows the order of their spatial deployment in the retinal cell population. Thus, it is extremely risky to try to correlate discontinuities or continuities in the retinal fiber projection to the tectum with a history of surgical manipulation of the retinotectal system. At best the map permits a correlation between the direction in which these locus specificities are deployed in the eye and the previous developmental history of the eye's orientation with respect to the body. Thus, the main limitation of the technique is that, in an experimental eye, it cannot assay the range of the position-dependent properties or tell whether the set of properties is complete, reduced, or augmented. However, it can provide information about the relative order with which the set of position-dependent properties has been spatially deployed in the retina. We have recently invented a technique which may make it possible to assay the range and the set of properties of the ganglion cells in an experimentally manipulated eye (Jacobson and Hunt, 1973). To do so we graft an experimental eye in the same eye socket as a normal eye at about embryonic stage 32. Both the normal and experimental eye project their optic nerve fibers into the same tectum. The normal eye serves as a standard since it is presumed to contain a full and normal set of position-dependent properties, and the mode of intercalation of the fibers from the two eyes into that part of the optic tectum that they share can provide quantitative information about the range and the set of properties of the retinal ganglion cells in the experimental eye. Such an assay has shown, for example, that eyes inverted _in situ_ contain a full set of position-dependent properties.

As the retinotectal mapping assay provides only limited information about the properties of retinal ganglion cells and none about the connections between retinal and tectal cells, it is necessary to use postsynaptic recording techniques as a crucial step towards an understanding of the expression of neuronal locus specificity (Skarf, 1973; Skarf and Jacobson, 1974). Without information about the transactions between the optic nerve fiber tips and the tectal cells which result in the formation of functional retinotectal synapses we stand no hope of understanding the expression of cellular mechanisms which determine how nerve fibers reach the proper places and how nerve fiber tips discriminate amongst potential postsynaptic cells. Although a beginning has been made in the postsynaptic analysis of retinotectal connectivity (Skarf, 1973; Skarf and Jacobson, 1974), the appropriate experiments have not been done which may show whether the formation of a retinotectal synapse occurs without reference to the other synapses in its vicinity (that is in a noncontextual mode) or whether retinotectal synaptogenesis is a contextual process in which many pre- and postsynaptic elements cooperate.

Returning again to the strategies that we have used for studying the genesis of position-dependent properties in the retinal ganglion cells, first we have to show that the position-dependent properties are truly dependent upon position in the retinal cell population and are not merely an expression of some temporal order in development such as the order of origin of retinal ganglion cells, the order of their differentiation, and the timing of the arrival of the retinal axons in the tectum. That the latter was not the case was shown in experiments in which eyes were either grafted from stage 32 embryos to the body wall for 30 days or explanted into tissue culture for ten days before being reimplanted in the orbit and allowed to form connections with the brain. These eyes formed normal retinotopically organized projections with orientations which were appropriate to the positions of the eyes in the original donors (Hunt and Jacobson, 1972a,b). When such an eye was allowed to compete with a normal eye during innervation of a single tectum both projected in register with no parts of the tectum being unshared. These experiments showed that the expression of locus specificities does not depend upon sequential order of arrival of nerve fibers from the eye into the tectum. It was then necessary to discover whether the position-dependence was derived from the position of the ganglion cell within the retinal field or was derived from the position of the eye on the body surface. For this purpose we transplanted a stage 28 eye rudiment on to the body wall of a stage 28 intermediate host in various orientations as is shown in Figure 2 (Hunt and Jacobson, 1972a). After the eye had developed to mid-stage 30 it was reintroduced to the orbit of a stage 39 carrier embryo and allowed to form connections with the brain. The resulting retinotectal projections were normally organized and were oriented in a position appropriate to the orientation of the eye on the body wall. When such an eye was allowed to compete with a normal eye in the innervation of a single tectum both eyes projected to the entire tectum with no area left unshared. The set of specificities in the experimental eye, which had spent its critical period on the body wall, was indistinguishable from the set of specificities in the normal eye. Therefore, the positional-dependence of locus specificity is derived not from some absolute position on the body surface but from the relative positions of the ganglion cells within the retinal field (Hunt and Jacobson, 1972a). Apparently then, the eye is not directly instructed by the embryo about its absolute position on the body, but merely uses the body as a source of positional cues for establishing properly aligned axes of its own.

Clearly the axial cues are not unique to the tissues surrounding the eye but are also available to an eye on the side of the body. This raises the possibility that the same cues may be used to align the axes of other organ rudiments such as the limb or the ears. Like the eye, those organ rudiments also acquire axial cues from the surrounding tissues which then participate in aligning the axes of the organ rudiment with the axes of the embryo (Harrison, 1921; 1945; Swett, 1937; Hall, 1939).

The next question that arises is whether the transition from the unspecified to the specified state involves stable and irreversible changes in the retinal cells or whether, in contrast, the change in the state of the system reflects changes in the extra-ocular conditions in the embryo. An example of the latter change might be the disappearance of axial cues required to reorganize retinal axes after eye rotation or transplantation of the eye. To test whether the transition which occurs at stage 29 to 31 involves irreversible changes in the eye or in the embryo, we back-grafted stage 31-32 right eyes into the enucleated right orbits of stage 28 embryos as shown in Figure 3 (Hunt and Jacobson, 1972b). When the eye was back-grafted in an inverted position the pattern of retinotectal connections which developed was retinotopically organized but inverted in both axes of the tectum. When the back-grafted eye was introduced into a stage 28 orbit in normal orientation, a normally oriented retinotectal projection invariably developed. These results show that the back-grafting procedures themselves did not alter the pattern of retinotectal connectivity and that a back-grafted stage 31-32 eye developed locus specificities from positional information obtained in the original donor orbit and failed to show the influence of its new position in the host orbit. The stage 31-32 eye is thus refractory to the same conditions which are capable of providing positional information to an unspecified eye in a stage 28 animal. In addition, we have tested the independent stability of the anteroposterior and dorsoventral axial components of locus specificity by back-grafting stage 31-32 left eyes into stage 28 right orbits. Such a transfer inverts one retinal axis only. In these instances the retinotectal projections developing from the back-grafted eye were inverted in one axis and normal in the other. The independent stability of the two axial components of locus specificity was confirmed in several cases in which eyes were back-grafted at stage 30, intermediate between specification in the two axes. Thus anteroposterior inversion of the retinotectal map resulted from back-grafting stage 30 right eyes, in an inverted orientation, into stage 28 right orbits.

These experiments provide strong evidence that the transition from the unspecified to the specified state involves stable and irreversible changes in the eyes between stages 29 and 32, but whether irreversible changes also occur in the embryo remains unknown. That the axial cues persist until stage 39 and are available to a stage 28 eye implanted into a stage 39 embryo was shown in the following experiment illustrated in Figure 4A. A stage 23 eye was transplanted in rotated position into a stage 28 host, allowed to traverse the critical period of that host, and then reimplanted into a stage 39 carrier embryo (Hunt and Jacobson, 1973). The reimplantation was done before the eye itself had reached its critical period. Such eyes always developed normal retinotectal projections regardless of their orientation in the final carrier embryo. These experiments show that the trigger mechanism for the transition from unspecified to specified state is not the sudden disappearance at stage 28 of the extraocular axial cues, which presumably participate in organizing the retinal axes and aligning them with the major axes of the body. Rather the trigger mechanisms are within the eye itself. That the transition during the critical period was not due to extraocular agents which transiently arise between stages 28 and 32 was shown in the following experiment. Unspecified eyes before stage 28 were transferred directly to carrier embryos between stages 32 and 39. In all cases, regardless of the orientation of the eye in the final carrier, a normally oriented retinotectal projection developed. Thus, a normal pattern of retinotectal projections developed from an eye which had never been in contact with an embryo at the critical stages of 28 to 32. These experiments eliminate a classical induction model of specification in which extraocular agents arise transiently during the critical period and instruct or specify an unspecified retinal cell population.

That the specification process does not involve instructive action on the part of the embryo but merely a transition from a reversible to an irreversible state is shown by the experiment shown in Figure 4B. Eye rediments from stage 22 to 25 embryos were cultured *in vitro* for periods of two to four days during which the eyes developed the features of stages 38 or 39 normal eyes. These mature explants were then reimplanted into stage 39 carrier embryos (Hunt and Jacobson, 1973). In these cases the resulting retinotectal maps were normal when the eye was in its normal orientation in the final carrier but when the eye was rotated the map was rotated to the same extent, showing that the locus specificities in the retinal ganglion cell population were derived from the original donor and were not altered in the final carrier. These experiments show that specification occurs in tissue culture in total isolation from the embryo and that the eye as early as stage 22 contains a set of reference axes properly aligned with the axes of the stage 22 embryo. The embryonic eye in the unspecified state before stage 28 possesses a stable but reversible set of axes. Whether these axes are physically the same as those that are present after stage 31 remains to be determined. However, it is certain that the specification process merely consists of a transition from a reversible but stable set of axes in the unspecified retina to a stable but irreversible set of retinal axes in the specified retina.

As specification occurs in isolation from the embryo it requires no instructive action from the tissues outside the eye. The change in the eye that renders the retinal cells refractory to the continuing influence of axial cues from the surrounding cues remains to be considered. The foregoing discussion has defined the changes of state through which the retinal cell population goes in the development of definitive locus specificities but it has left open the question of cellular mechanisms. We would like to elucidate the cellular mechanisms of (1) deployment of position-dependent properties in the retinal cell population, (2) substitution of new retinal axes after eye inversion, and (3) expression of the properties as locus specificities during the morphogenesis of the retinotectal projection. One limitation of the experiments that have been described is that, while they are able to define the state of the total retinal cell population in the intact eye, they do not show the state of individual retinal cells. An additional problem arises from the fact that at stages 29 to 30 the retina contains about 500 cells but the locus specificities are determined not only for the cells that are then present but for all the retinal ganglion cells (about 500,000) that will ultimately develop in the adult eye (Jacobson, 1968a,b). Because we operate on the embryos but only assay the locus specificities in the adult eye, we do not know when the final set of locus specificities developes. The retina grows by addition of new cells at its margin (Glücksmann, 1940) where a population of retinal stem cells persists throughout embryonic and larval development. The question then arises whether the nerve cells acquire specificity from the stem cells as a result of cell lineage, or whether, in addition or exclusively, they acquire specificity by interacting with other cells. If the former is true, how do the stem cells pass on the specificity to their progeny? If the latter, do the newborn nerve cells interact with other cells within the eye or with cells outside the eye, or with both?

Another problem arises because nerve cells die during normal retinal histogenesis (Glücksmann, 1940; 1951; 1965). How is the pattern of deployment of position-dependent properties in the retinal cell population affected by cell death? Other unanswered questions are: why do some neurons die and others survive; is cell death random or selective; do ganglion cells die before, during or after the arrival of their axons in the tectum; and does ganglion cell death play any part in sorting of retinal fibers in the tectum?

At present, our only clues to a solution of these problems are certain correlations between retinal histogenesis and the genesis of locus specificities in the retinal ganglion cell population. First, the retinal ganglion cells that are born in the central region of the retina cease DNA synthesis at stages 29 to 31 (Jacobson, 1967; 1968b) and it seems likely that changes in their developmental programs accompanying their withdrawal which initiates the transition from the unspecified to the specified state. One may, with some confidence, propose the hypothesis that in many different neuronal populations the change from the unspecified to the specified state occurs as nerve cells become postmitotic, that is, at the time of their birth. One cause of the change of state that occurs at that stage of the nerve cell's development, may be that the postmitotic cell uncouples from the stem cell, and thus loses the capacity to interact with the stem cell population. Apparently developing nerve cells, when grafted to another position, can acquire new position-dependent properties only if they can couple functionally with neighboring cells. The locus specificities of the grafted cells then develop in accord with their new positions. However, if the graft itself cannot communicate with neighboring cells, its locus specificities are derived from the original position before grafting. Intercellular communication of the type envisaged here appears to be dependent upon specialized cellular junctions (Loewenstein, 1968; 1970) that provide pathways for the movement of ions and small molecules between the cells of the embryo (Loewenstein, 1968; 1970; Sheridan, 1968; Warner, 1970). Intercellular junctions of the gap junction variety have been found ubiquitously between the cells of the embryonic retina of Xenopus before stage 29 (while the retina is composed of mitotically active stem cells), but disappear from the retinal cells in the center of the retina during the critical stages 29 to 32 (as the first retinal nerve cells, destined to become ganglion cells, withdraw from the mitotic cycle), and at later stages persist only between the cells at the retinal margins (which remain mitotically active) (Dixon and Cronley-Dillon, 1972). Our experiments (Loewenstein, Rose and Jacobson, unpublished) have demonstrated the passage of fluorescent-labeled molecules between cells of the embryonic retina before stage 30, but have shown that such intercellular communication is impeded or absent at later stages of development of the retina. Therefore, it seems that the change of state at the critical period involves withdrawal of retinal cells from the mitotic cycle and concomitant uncoupling of the postmitotic nerve cells from the rest of the retinal cell population. After uncoupling from the retinal population the nerve cell is characterized by a stable and irreversible position-dependent property which results in the development of definitive locus specificity. Development of this position-dependent specificity enables the young nerve cell to extend its outgrowing axon on the proper pathway, predisposes that axon to terminate at a specific position in the brain and to form synaptic connections selectively with particular nerve cells. Therefore, the position-dependence of the nerve cell is expressed at several stages of its developmental program. How this control of the nerve cell's position occurs in terms of cellular mechanisms remains an unsolved problem of developmental neurobiology.

REFERENCES

Dixon, J. S. and Cronly-Dillon, J.R. (1972). J. Embryol. Exp. Morphol. 28, 659.

Glücksmann, A. (1940). Brit. J. Ophthalmol. 24, 153.

Glücksmann, A. (1951). Biol. Revs. 26, 59.

Glücksmann, A. (1965). Arch. Biol. (Liege) 76, 419.

Hall, E.K. (1939). J. Exp. Zool. 82, 173.

Harrison, R.G. (1921). J. Exp. Zool. 32, 1.

Harrison, R.G. (1945). Trans. Conn. Acad. Arts Sci. 36,277.

Hunt, R.K. and Jacobson, M. (1972a). Proc. Nat. Acad. Sci. U.S.A. 69, 780.

Hunt, R.K. and Jacobson, M. (1972b). Proc. Nat. Acad. Sci. U.S.A. 69, 2860.

Hunt, R.K. and Jacobson, M. (1973). Proc. Nat. Acad. Sci. U.S.A. 70, 507.

Jacobson, M. (1967). Science 155, 1106.

Jacobson, M. (1968a). Develop. Biol. 17, 202.

Jacobson, M. (1968b). Develop. Biol. 17, 219.

Jacobson, M. and Hunt, R.K. (1973). Sci. Amer. 228, 26.

Loewenstein, W.R. (1968). Persp. Biol. Med. 11, 260.

Loewenstein, W.R. (1970). Sci. Amer. 222, 78.

Sheridan, J.D. (1968). J. Cell Biol. 37, 650.

Skarf, B. (1973). Brain Res. 51, 352.

Skarf, B. and Jacobson, M. (1974). Brain Res. (in press).

Sperry, R.W. (1950). In "Genetic Neurology" (P. Weiss, ed.) pp. 232-239, Univ. Chicago Press, Chicago.

Sperry, R.W. (1963). Proc. Nat. Acad. Sci. U.S.A. 50, 703.

Swett, F.H. (1937). Quart. Rev. Biol. 12, 322.

Warner, A.E. (1970). J. Physiol. (London) 210, 150.

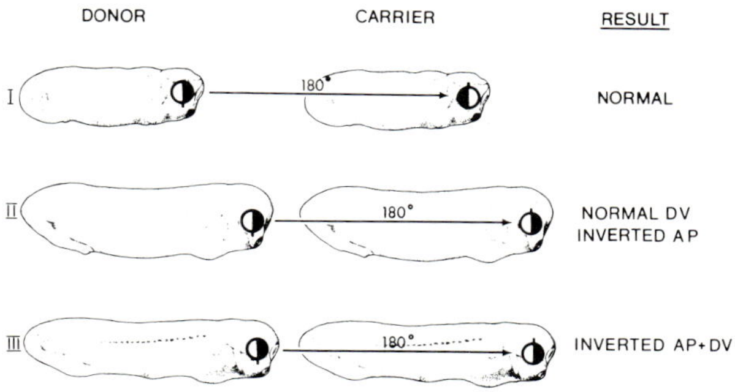

Fig. 1 Critical period is at stages 29 to 31: (I) If the eye is inverted at stage 28, the retinotectal map is normal; (II) if the eye is inverted at stage 30, the retinotectal map is inverted in the anteroposterior retinal axis; (III) eye inversion at stage 31 or later, completely inverts the retinotectal projection.

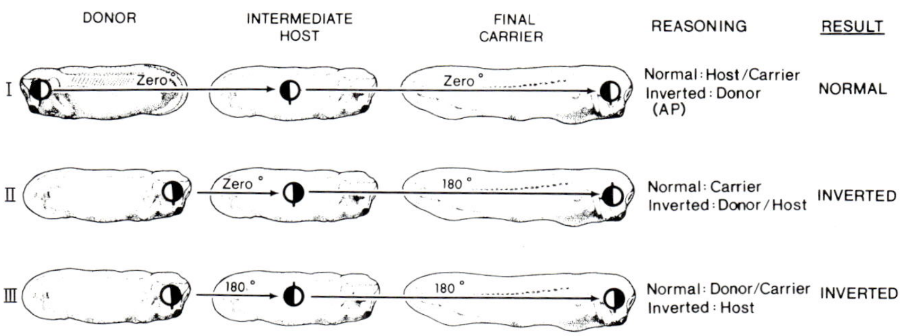

Fig. 2 Positional cues are obtained by a stage 28 eye grafted to the flank of a stage 28 host, where the eye traverses its critical period and is then grafted to the orbit of a final carrier at stage 32 to 34. The retinotectal projection, mapped in the carrier, shows that the retinal locus specificities originated when the eye was on the flank of the intermediate host.

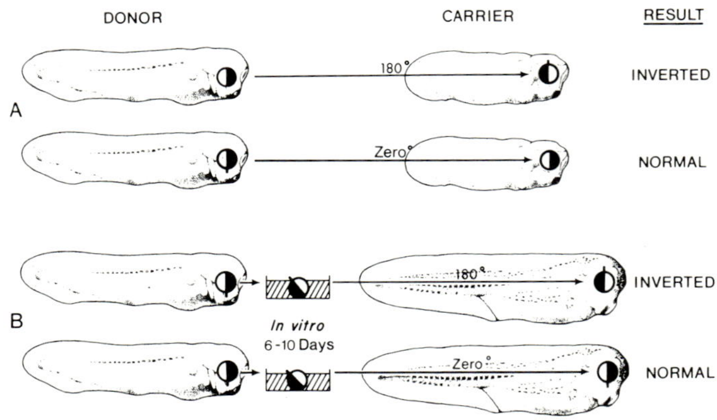

Fig. 3A A specified eye (stage 31) back-grafted to a stage 28 carrier does not realign its axes but completes the development of the retinotectal projection in correspondence with the orientation of the eye in the final carrier.

Fig. 3B Isolation of the specified stage 31 eye in tissue culture for 6 to 10 days does not alter the developmental program which is completed when the eye is grafted in the orbit of a stage 39 carrier. The retinotectal projection corresponds with the orientation of the eye in the final carrier.

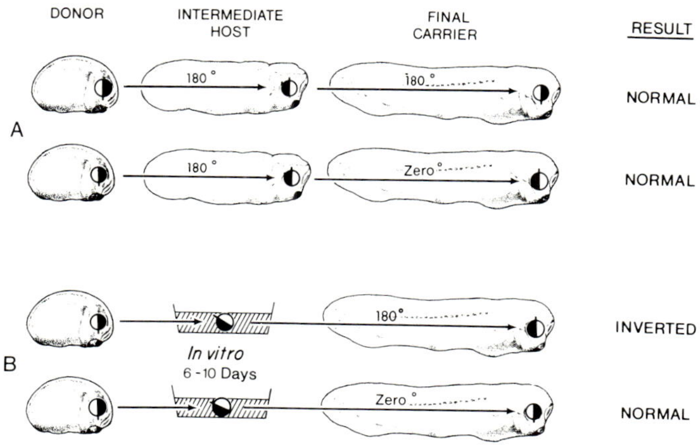

Fig. 4A Trigger for specification at the critical stages 29 to 31 is in the eye and positional cues persist thereafter in the embryo. An eye from a stage 22 embryo is not specified prematurely when grafted to a stage 28 intermediate host, but the critical stage is attained according to the eye's own developmental schedule, which occurs in the eye after it is grafted to a stage 32 carrier.

Fig. 4B That an eye can be specified *in vitro* and then successfully complete its developmental program when grafted to a stage 32 to 39 carrier shows: (a) that specification does not require instruction from tissues outside the eye; (b) that a stage 22 eye contains positional infomation necessary for later development of retinal locus specificity; (c) that position-dependent properties in the eye are stable for 6-10 days in the absence of interactions between eye and embryo.

AGING OF THE VERTEBRATE BRAIN

Harold Brody

Department of Anatomical Sciences
State University of New York at Buffalo
Buffalo, New York 14214

When compared with other scientific disciplines, the study of aging may be considered to be of recent origin and, as characterizes new fields of inquiry, the descriptive phase is to a great extent still operative. Systematic observations of differences associated with age and used for data gathering and orderly collections of observed facts are a necessity in systematizing knowledge and yet unknown principles and laws governing aging.

A prerequisite for studies of the biochemical, physiological and immunological relationships of aging in the central nervous system must be an understanding of the morphological changes in structures essential to normal nervous system functioning.

In a study of the brains of 47 vertebrate species, Dayan (1971) attempted to relate some indicators of aging in the human with the appearance in other vertebrates. In doing so, he emphasized a basic difficulty in discussing aging in organisms other than man. Certainly there is little agreement among investigators in this field as to what is a senile animal. A personal observation would be that there must be an agreement reached on a world-wide level as to what constitutes an old animal and that this interpretation needs to be adhered to for the study of aging in every species, be it vertebrate or invertebrate so that some consistency can develop in the interpretation of findings.

As noted in other organs of man, the brain undergoes certain atrophic changes. The dura becomes adherent to the underlying tissue while the leptomeninges, the pia-arachnoid layer, thickens and becomes opaque in appearance. The arachnoid villi also demonstrate fibrosis and calcification.

In contrast with these findings in man, Dayan (1971) found that no consistent trend appeared in the external appearance of the brains of 139 animals and birds of 47 different species, although in the old giraffe, parrot, red deer and some dogs, the leptomeninges appeared gray and semi-opaque. However, there was a great variation between members of the same species.

Brain weight has been studied by a number of workers (Boyd, 1895; Pearl, 1905; Appel and Appel, 1942a, 1942b; Pakkenberg and Voigt, 1964) who demonstrate a decrease in brain weight of some 90-100 grams by 70 years of age.

While there is a generalized atrophy evident on gross examination of the cerebral hemispheres, this is particularly so in the frontal, parietal and temporal areas. The gyri become more narrowed and the sulci widened. This cortical shrinkage is accompanied by an atrophy of the underlying white matter. In addition, there is a dilatation of the ventricular system, and with the widening of the sulci, an increase in the subarachnoid space surrounding the hemispheres. As early as 1928, Inukai, in explaining the loss of brain weight with age, attributed this to a loss of neurons, although no data was presented to support this idea. Hodge (1894) had reported a decrease in cells in spinal ganglia between newborn and the 92-year-old and Gardner (1940) reported more than a 30% decrease in posterior root ganglion neurons between the 5th and 9th decades.

Ellis (1919) and Harms (1927) had also noted a decrease of approximately 25% in the number of Purkinje cells in the human cerebellum. Dayan (1971), in his vertebrate study, reported a "readily apparent" loss of Purkinje cells which was diffusely distributed throughout all lobes of the cerebellum. While no neurons were noted in the process of degeneration, it appeared that fallout had occurred to account for the presence of empty baskets in 28 of the 74 animals and birds in which the cerebellum was examined. Quantitation was not performed on these specimens attesting to the fact that the cell decrease was considered quite obvious by this investigator. No marked loss of neurons was noted in the cerebral cortex, although thickening of the outer molecular layer with age in older animals with younger aged controls made it seem likely that some neuron loss had occurred. Critchley (1942) and

Riese (1946) reported a seemingly greater loss of cells occurring in layer 3 (the outer pyramidal layer) of the cerebral cortex of man, although these conclusions were not based on a quantitative approach and were observed in brains from a state hospital population. By preparing sonificated suspensions of mouse brain, Johnson and Erner (1972) have found a decrease of the neuron population to one-third of its original size in 29-month-old animals.

Considering the often profound changes which occur in behavior and mental ability as one ages, our attention has been directed to the cerebral cortex (Brody, 1955). Tissues have been obtained from individuals who had not demonstrated any pathology related to the nervous system and specimens were removed between one-half hour and 4 hours after death. They were perfused with 10% formol-saline solution by injection through the internal carotid and vertebral arteries. Ten micron paraffin sections from blocks of tissue of specific cortical areas (fig. 1) were stained with cresyl echt violet. A standard Howard type eyepiece disc was orientated so that the upper line was placed along the pial surface of the cortex within a sulcus, in order that cells could be counted without the risk of duplicate counts, as could occur were the cortex on the dome surface of the gyrus to be used as a source area. Examining the section under high dry magnification, the neurons in each row of six squares lying parallel to the surface were counted. When all cells within the 36 squares of the reticule had been counted, the next deeper area was counted by shifting the section, until the entire depth of the cortex had been examined. The section was then shifted to count nerve cells in the next adjacent column again beginning at the pial surface. Five columns were counted in this way. The total number of cells in these five columns would provide us with the cell population for this particular area of cortex. To determine the distribution of cells within the layers of that cortical region, the number of cells within each two adjacent columns of the reticule parallel to the surface can be totalled. This strip of cortex equal to two layers of the reticule or 75μ extends through the five columns of cells. The size of this strip remains constant, though the region of cortex changes as one descends through the depth of the cortex. The cell number within each of these 2 layers can then be graphed against the depth below the cortical surface (fig. 2), and the graph produced is a profile of the cell population arranged in layers so that those layers of the cerebral cortex containing a larger number of cells (2, 4 and 6) may be distinguished from those layers with a lesser number (1, 3 and 5). These determinations in a number of cortical areas demonstrate that cerebral cortex does not show an equal decrease in cell number in all regions, but there is evidence that neuronal decrease involves certain areas to a greater extent than others and one is impressed with the possibility that this may account for the more specific involvement of certain functions to a greater extent than others. In some earlier studies, the greatest decrease in cell number occurred in the superior temporal gyrus, to a lesser extent in the precentral gyrus, followed by decreasing but significant cell loss in the visual cortex and postcentral gyrus. The cell number in the superior temporal cortex of the 90-year-old indicated a decrease of approximately one-third of the number reported for the 19-year-old person. Note should be taken of the fact that the cortex of the infant shows a higher cell content within a unit area than does the same sized area in the adult brain. Nerve cells being post-mitotic, do not increase in cell number after birth. Conel (1947) has demonstrated that except for the striate area or primary visual cortex, cortical width increased with further development, due to increasing length of glial and nerve cell processes, increase in myelin and the increase in the quantity and size of other elements such as blood vessels. Due to these factors, the number of nerve cells per unit area in the mature cortex is much less than the cell number of the same size area in the infant cortex. After the 16- to 21-year-old age group, by which time the brain has reached its maximum size, so that this period can be considered as the base time, the evidence indicates a decrease in cell number with increasing age.

Our studies have been extended into the superior frontal gyrus with examination of specimens between the 5th and 9th decades. Table 1 indicates the age distribution and the number of cells counted in each specimen of the superior frontal gyrus. While within groups there may be some differences in cell number, there is, in general, a clustering by decades and an obvious downward trend. Fig. 3 shows that the most marked change occurs during the 5th decade after which the decrease in cell number continues, although at a decreased rate.

This decrease occurs in all cortical layers, but is most marked in layers 2 and 4, the external and internal granule layers where the Golgi type II short axoned cells are characteristic of the associational cells of the human cerebral cortex.

While these studies of changes in cell number in the cerebral cortex may be of great significance, one must wonder about the relationship of age in other regions of the central nervous system. Van Buskirk in 1945 had found no cell loss in the motor nucleus of the facial nerve and Konigsmark and Murphy (1970, 1972) found no difference with age in the ventral cochlear nucleus. Several specific nuclear groups in the brain stem have been examined and compared with cerebral cortex. One may examine the brain stem with greater ease than cortex since specific nuclear groups may be easily identified, serial sections cut and total cell counts taken throughout the entire length of the structure. The nucleus of the inferior olive in the medulla oblongata has been examined from the prenatal period to 89 years in 10μ cresyl echt violet sections counted in serial fashion. Table 2 presents the ages and sex of 18 specimens. The measured length relates to the measurement in the gross specimen while the calculated length which is more precise was obtained from microscopic sections measuring the distance between the presence of the most caudal and rostral cell in the main nucleus of the inferior olive. Shrinkage occurring in preparation of the tissue was not calculated, but all specimens were prepared in the same way. Also presented is the total cell count estimated by counting all cells with nucleoli in every tenth section and multiplying by a factor of 10. While the inferior olive changes in size from 8mm on day zero to a postnatal mean of 13.16mm in calculated length, the number of cells in the postnatal period to 89 years shows no significant change in number with a mean of 363,784 cells.

Fig. 4 illustrates the cell distribution within the length of the main inferior olivary nucleus of the newborn and 3-day-old infant, while fig. 5 shows a comparison of cell distribution within the length of the olive in a 32- and 65-year-old. These graphs demonstrate a similarity in length and cell distribution in two young and two adult specimens.

However (fig. 6), when a 3-month-old is compared with

a 9-year-old, although the difference in cell number is not significant, the infant illustrates a marked increase in cell density with a packing of cells into a much more restricted area. This also illustrates the importance of performing full serial counts when it is possible to do so. Counting the cells on a single section through the middle of the inferior olive of these respective specimens would have presented an erroneous impression of a marked cell loss in the 9-year-old specimen.

The presence of lipofuscin pigment within the aging nerve cell has been mentioned as a factor which interferes with cell metabolism, eventually resulting in the death of the cell. The fact that there is no significant neuron loss in the inferior olive is of additional interest since lipofuscin pigment makes its first appearance in the 3-month-old specimen and by 38 years of age, is present to the extent that 84% of inferior olivary cells contain a large enough amount of lipofuscin so as to occupy the entire parenchyma of the cell, pushing the nucleus into an eccentric position. By 70 years of age, 100% of these cells contain this excessive amount of the pigment without any significant change in cell number (fig. 7).

In further studies of the human brain stem, we have concerned ourselves with an evaluation of the nuclei of the trochlear and abducens nerves as well as the locus caeruleus. For these structures, specimens have been examined from newborn to 86 years of age. The trochlear nucleus increases in size from 1.3mm in the newborn to approximately 2.0 in the adult, while the mean cell count of 2,100 (with a range of 1,810 to 2,400 cells) shows no significant change in cell number with increasing age. The abducens nucleus, whose length almost doubles between newborn and adult, also shows no significant change in cell number (with a mean for all ages of 6,500 cells). Only in the locus caeruleus have we been able to show a significant difference in cell number, although this has not appeared until the 9th decade. We are now examining this question in additional specimens, since this finding is the first noted change in cell number within a brain stem structure.

From these studies with the help of my collaborators, Dr. Reneé Monagle (deceased) and Dr. N. Vijayashankar and reports in the literature, there is, I believe, good evidence to indicate a difference in the effects of age upon cerebral cortex as compared with brain stem structures in the human. As other areas of the central nervous system are examined, it is probable that differential rates of cell loss varying from extensive to minimal or null will be determined. It does not seem reasonable to assume that all parts of the central nervous system should be affected equally during aging. Certainly evidence is available to illustrate the specific sensitivity of certain areas to pathological conditions and the stress of aging ought to, we believe, involve certain brain areas to a greater extent than others.

REFERENCES

Appel, F.W. and Appel, E.M. (1942a). Human Biol. 14, 48.

Appel, F.W. and Appel, E.M. (1942b). Human Biol. 14, 235.

Boyd, R. (1895). In "Quain's Anatomy" (E.A. Schafer and G.D. Thane, eds.), Vol. III, Part 1, 10th ed., pp. 219, Longmans and Green, London.

Brody, H. (1955). J. Comp. Neurol. 102, 511.

Conel, J.L. (1947). "The Postnatal Development of the Human Cerebral Cortex", Vol. III. The cortex of the three month old infant. Howard Univ. Press, Boston.

Critchley, MacDonald (1942). In "Problems of Ageing" (E.V. Cowdry, ed.), 2nd ed., pp. 518-534, Williams and Wilkins, Baltimore.

Dayan, A.D. (1971). Brain 94, 31.

Ellis, R.S. (1919). J. Comp. Neurol. 30, 229.

Gardner, E.D. (1940). Anat. Record 77, 529.

Harms, J.W. (1927). Zool. Anz. 74, 249.

Hodge, C.F. (1894). J. Physiol. 17, 129.

Inukai, T. (1928). J. Comp. Neurol. 45, 1.

Johnson, H.A. and Erner, S. (1972). Exp. Gerontol. 7, 111.

Konigsmark, B.W. and Murphy, E.A. (1970). Nature 228, 1355.

Konigsmark, B.W. and Murphy, E.A. (1972). J. Neuropathol. Exp. Neurol. 31, 304.

Pakkenberg, H. and Voigt, J. (1964). Acta Anat. 56, 297.

Pearl, R. (1905). Biometrika 4, 13.

Riese, W. (1946). J. Neuropathol. Exp. Neurol. 5, 160.

Van Buskirk, C. (1945). J. Comp. Neurol. 82, 303.

TABLE 1

Specimens used in the study of the relationship of age to nerve cell number in the superior frontal gyrus of the human male.

Age in years	Superior frontal gyrus Frontal pole
41	1,720
43	1,640
45	1,666
46	1,680
50	1,115
54	1,220
54	1,204
57	1,115
60	1,053
66	1,085
66	1,218
68	1,015
73	994
75	910
77	935
83	802
86	775
87	901

TABLE 2

Summary of sizes and cell number in the main nucleus of the inferior olive

Specimen Number	Age[1] Sex[2]	Measured Length in mm	Calculated Length in mm	Total Cell Count
1	23 wp-F	6 mm	6.0 mm	233,360
2	24 wp-F	6 mm	4.9 mm	247,240
3	30 wp-M	8 mm	6.8 mm	300,790
4	34 wp-M	8 mm	7.0 mm	346,850
5	0 day-F	11 mm	8.0 mm	330,610
6	3 days-M	13 mm	8.5 mm	327,330
7	3 mos.-M	12 mm	8.5 mm	380,460
8	9 yrs.-F	16 mm	17.9 mm	370,370
9	12 yrs.-F	15 mm	12.0 mm	366,100
10	19 yrs.-M	17 mm	13.9 mm	368,570
11	32 yrs.-M	15 mm	14.8 mm	364,930
12	44 yrs.-M	16 mm	13.9 mm	355,560
13	56 yrs.-M	15 mm	14.8 mm	389,610
14	65 yrs.-M	16 mm	13.7 mm	376,420
15	73 yrs.-M	18 mm	16.0 mm	405,580
16	77 yrs.-M	18 mm	14.4 mm	358,920
17	82 yrs.-M	17 mm	14.2 mm	317,600
18	89 yrs.-M	17 mm	13.6 mm	380,920
Prenatal Mean		7 mm	6.18mm	282,060
Postnatal Mean		19.1mm	13.16mm	363,784

[1] wp = weeks prenatal
[2] F = female; M = male

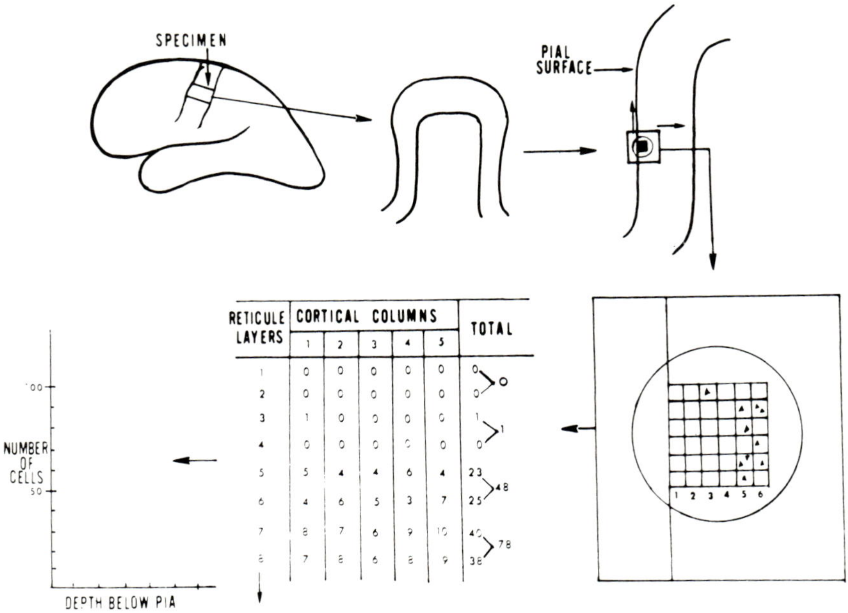

RETICULE LAYERS	CORTICAL COLUMNS 1	2	3	4	5	TOTAL
1	0	0	0	0	0	0 } 0
2	0	0	0	0	0	0
3	1	0	0	0	0	1 } 1
4	0	0	0	0	0	0
5	5	4	4	6	4	23 } 48
6	4	6	5	3	7	25
7	8	7	6	9	10	40 } 78
8	7	8	6	8	9	38

Fig. 1. From a block of tissue of a specific cortical area, sections (after staining) are examined for cell number with a Howard type reticule. A graph relating cell number to depth of the cortex may be constructed.

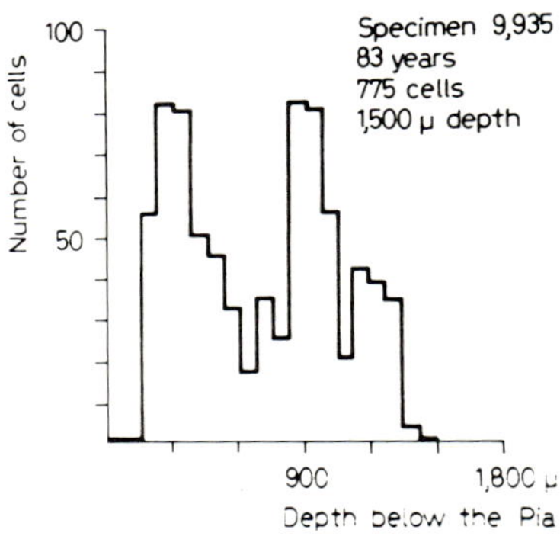

Fig. 2. Distribution of nerve cells in the superior frontal gyrus of an 83-year-old male.

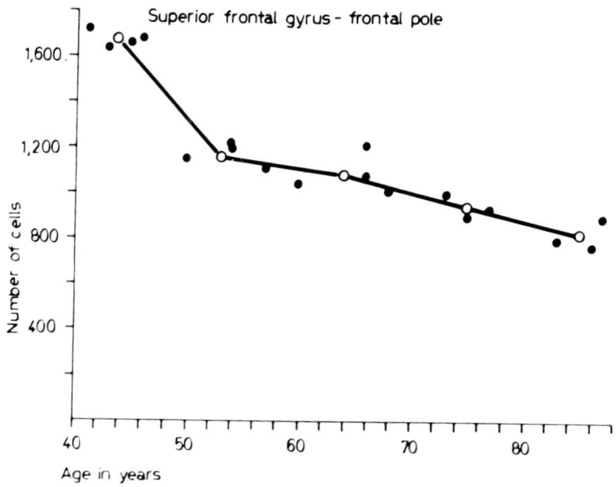

Fig. 3. The relationship of age to cell number in the superior frontal gyrus.

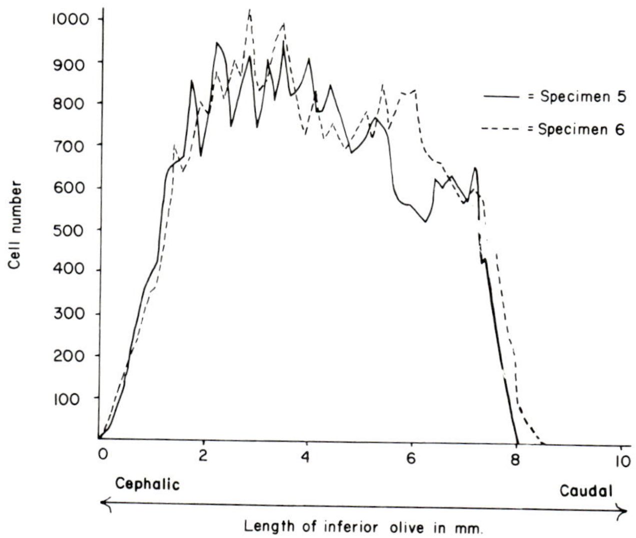

Fig. 4. The distribution of cells within the entire length of the inferior olivary nucleus of a newborn (specimen 5) and a 3-day-old (specimen 6).

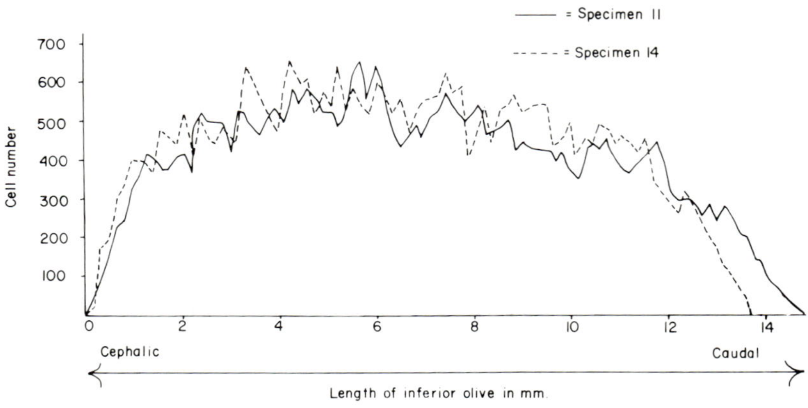

Fig. 5. The distribution of cells within the entire length of the inferior olivary nucleus of a 32-year-old (specimen 11) and a 65-year-old (specimen 14).

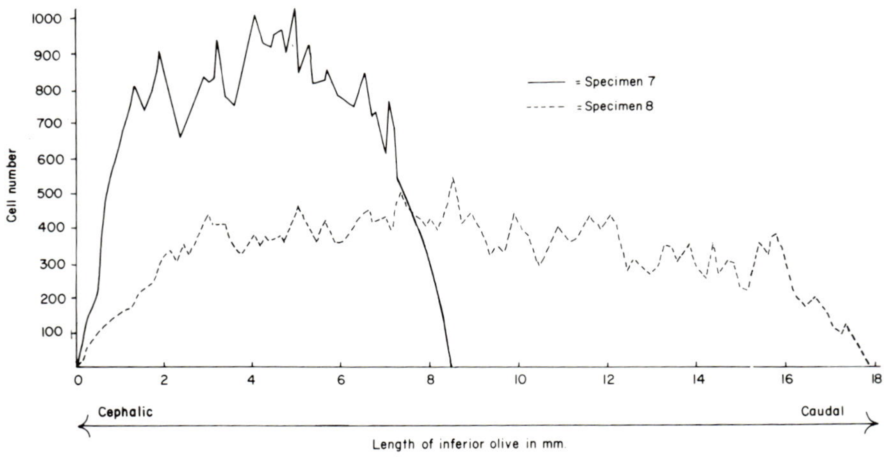

Fig. 6. A comparison of cell distribution within the human inferior olivary nucleus of a 3-month-old and a 9-year-old.

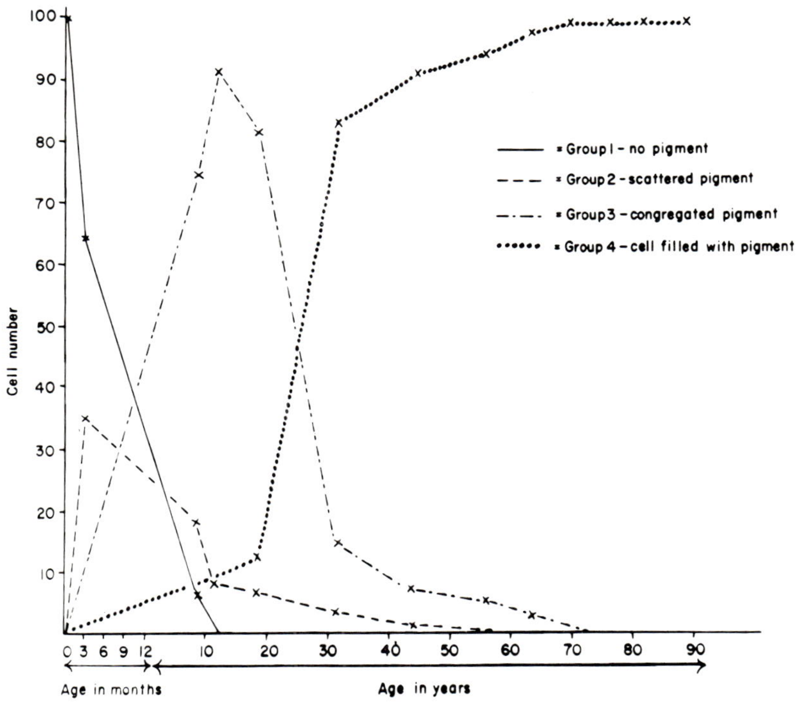

Fig. 7. Distribution of lipofuscin pigment within the cells of the inferior olivary nucleus.

INSULTS TO THE BRAIN. DIFFERENTIAL EFFECTS OF AGING

Frederick Richardson, M.D., M.R.C.P.

University of Miami
School of Medicine
Miami, Florida 33152

The observations made in clinical medicine are inherently subject to many potential errors because of the number of variables present in any given situation. However, nature itself is so orderly in its schemas and hierarchical organization that repeated observation of spontaneously occurring experiments in nature may lead to valid scientific hypotheses which are strengthened, modified or refuted as further clinical or experimental observations are made and substantiated.

Each bona fide hypothesis when based on a valid clinical observation is not worthless if it brings forth thoughtful comment which improves the interpretation of the original observation or leads to a new concept. Of critical importance in discussion of any disease state or change is the appreciation that the host or patient response to an acute or chronic lesion may vary for reasons that are little understood. Without diminishing or belittling the importance of accurate diagnosis or description of the lesion, the patient's adaptative and individual response to the lesion is more important in the field of clinical developmental medicine. Some have implied that the well-being of soma determines the nature and course of action of psyche - however, we are all aware of the converse - the critical importance of the vigilant mind to the optional function and purposes of the body.

Nowhere is this more apparent in general terms than in the complex processes of maturation and aging. One problem is to define what is meant by aging in man versus the concept of maturation. Intellectual maturity in man seems to imply a continuing process from one level of function to another and more complex level achieved through exposure, attention to and learning from conscious experience from which a distillate of knowledge comes. Tennyson has written "knowledge comes but wisdom lingers" - would it were always so. Man is a composite of cellular systems which subserve the total function and we have all witnessed deleterious effect of an insult either so massive or so exquisitely matched to the system it damages (as with carbon monoxide poisoning) that we can observe destruction of selective functions, mechanisms or a part of the brain without seriously aging or killing the host. I use the term host as there is frequently an individual variation in response to a disease or insult which is host-dependent and may well be host-system-dependent. Thus the frequent response to damage such as extrapyramidal disease may be dependent on such factors as whether or not it is part of a generalized atherosclerotic picture of Parkinson's Disease in an old man (Blackwood _et al._, 1963; Holmes, 1968), Wilson's Disease in the young (Shiraki, 1968), the delayed and insidious onset in the mature adult of the dread residuum of youthful encephalitis, or athetosis due to hypoxia in the perinatal period (Windle, 1958; Környey, 1963; Malamud, 1963).

The progression of disease of the nervous system over a period of years may pose an interesting clinical problem in that neurological function may not be related in a straightforward way to anticipated anotomical or pathological findings. An example is the lack of relationship clinically in peroneal muscular atrophy to the extensive spinal cord lesions often found pathologically. The patient's spinal cord may show gross and widespread damage involving many tracts whereas all that manifested clinically over a period of many years was a gradual and insidious onset of a slowly progressive disorder limited to muscular wasting and weakness for which adaptation and compensation has taken place (Blackwood _et al._, 1963).

In the study of infants and children much of the time and effort spent in the past has been directed to observation of development and maturation of gross motor abilities and psychological responses. The considerable variability in developmental observations from patient to patient, while of importance, has been of little or no predictive value in the individual. For example, very few of us would be prepared to base a serious estimate of a child's intellectual potential upon the age at which he took his first steps - the multiple variables from child to child even within the same family are so disparate that, in an attempt to better define dysfunction, more specific attention has been given to sense modality defects and the psychological measurement of memory, learning abilities and coding skills. The persistence of minimal cerebral function in a child, manifested behaviorally or neurologically, warrants a thorough assestment of neuropsychological function and the effect on performance and behavior (Paine, 1962; Birch, 1964).

Disturbance of both motor and psychological function may persist. An interesting example is the persistence of involuntary movement due to impaired development of inhibitory mechanisms. The ultimate effect of any insult appears to be related to the level of development and is thus age-dependent.

Mature or immature newborn infants may show spontaneous, delicate, slow, purposeless motor movements of the fingers and hands (Prechtl and Beintema, 1964). These are readily interrupted by a loud, sudden sound producing a startle reflex, with sudden outward-upward extension of the arms, fingers flexed with simultaneous flexion of the legs at the hips and knees. If the head is moved during the startle reflex, a Moro "Unklammerung" extensor reflex is also elicited due to labyrinthine stimulation associated with a deep neck reflex (Peiper, 1961; André-Thomas _et al._, 1960).

The persistence of the Moro response after the age of three months is a warning signal as to the possible presence of central nervous system damage. Similarly, persistence of a strong infant grasp reflex may be indicative of brain damage as is the failure to extinguish the startle reflex in the presence of quickly repetetive stimuli.

As part of the process of normal maturation, the infant enters a predominantly extrapyramidal period of choreoathetoid movements which are increased by almost any stimulation especially excitement, including the excitement of a purposive voluntary movement such as trying to hit or kick a rattle. We have all seen the 4-month infant, when excited, go through a veritable paroxysm of exaggerated reactive choreic jerky movements of short duration. They not infrequently accompany the normal (for age) but prolonged smile which can be readily elicited from an alert, happy infant even at the relatively mature age of one year. The smile is broad, exaggerated, prolonged, and often accompanied by an involuntary rotary jerking movement of the head (Richardson, 1965).

In an infant this is to be anticipated and is not out of place as it would be in a child of two years or in an adult. The involuntary jerky movements disappear naturally soon after the end of the first year of life as normal inhibitory mechanisms continue to develop, making purposeful voluntary movements easier, quicker and more accurate. Inhibition of many of the movements described could equally well be related to associated maturation of the inhibitory mechanisms of the cerebellum and its connections providing a continuous ongoing correction of movements (Eccles, 1973). Persistence of these movements or continued exaggeration of normal movement suggests impaired development of normal inhibitory mechanisms that control the quality of voluntary movements and this may lead into the picture of infantile cerebral palsy of the extrapyramidal type such as that seen following severe hemolytic jaundice of the newborn.

The cerebral control of movement in the mammalian brain and adaptation to insults in the developmental period is still poorly documented in contrast to studies of mature mammalian brain such as those of Sherrington (1961), and Denny-Brown (1966). As Eccles (1968) has pointed out, "The nervous system does not simply develop linearly in all directions, many things grow and regress".....at one and the same time.

In young children it is not uncommon to find hemiathetosis associated with the major picture of hemiparesis sometimes accompanied also by a sensory defect, (e.g., Case #837086, JHH, F.R.). I discussed the findings in several cases with Dr. Frank Ford (1960) at Johns Hopkins University some years ago, and he made the observation that, in his experience, in early lesions of the pyramidal tract associated with infantile hemiplegia, there is often found a small and underdeveloped corpus striatum on the ipsilateral side. This experiment in nature has been witnessed often enough to emphasize in a simple way the importance of <u>interdependence of functionally related</u> systems during development and what I term their <u>sympathetic vulnerability</u>, particularly during periods of rapid cellular growth and functional maturation.

It is well known that damage to the brain during the neonatal and perinatal period may leave little in the way of scarring or gliosis. The residual defect, if any, can be characterized by smaller number of cells, smaller cells or their complete absence. There is no "footprint" of scarring or gliosis such as may be seen in the mature brain (Johnson, 1972). In contrast, Brierley (1971) has emphasized that in the mature primate ischaemic alterations after a hypoxic episode are occasionally recognizable after a survival of only one hour. In the developmental period when human or animal lesions are due to hypoglycemia, or anoxia, the end result is, as one would expect, frequently indistinguishable one from the other.

This would appear to be a characteristic response of the immature growing brain, when interference with essential cellular (mitochondrial) utilization of the glucose oxygen substrate takes place. However, the lack of growth of systems anatomically and functionally related to the damaged area (sympathetic vulnerability) may be of some importance in determination of the timing and nature of the insult.

To return to the maturation of extrapyramidal control of movement, just as it appeared to be fairly characteristic that Parkinsonism may develop in young adults following encephalitis lethargica, or the insult of carbon monoxide poisoning, it appears that the responses to severe concussion of the brain are different at the age levels of infancy, childhood, adolescence and adulthood.

In a study conducted some years ago at Johns Hopkins of children and adolescents who had recovered from protracted coma (Richardson, 1963), concerned primarily with the intellectual and behavioral sequelae of coma and post-traumatic amnesia following severe acceleration concussion, as defined by Denny-Brown and Russell (1941), there appeared to be several age-dependent effects in the physical and neurological responses as well as clearly defined patterns of behavioral and intellectual sequelae.

The serious stresses on the brain in acceleration concussion are due to excessive acceleration and violent deceleration. The brain's own inertia, under these circumstances, causes severe internal strains and stresses often with shearing of neurones most commonly at or near the junction between white and grey matter. This is increased by the different densities of these two tissues (Holborn,

1945; Pudenz and Shelden, 1946).

In those who survive, the speed and degree of recovery is related directly to age:

Infants and children up to 4 years old, exposed to acceleration concussion with loss of consciousness usually recover rapidly and completely or they die quickly of acute cerebral edema. Prolonged vegitative survival in this young group is virtually unknown. Further studies by Black (1973) also corroborate this finding.

Children between 5 and 12 years make the best recovery even following protracted coma of several weeks. Prolonged post-traumatic amnesia and decerebrate rigidity vegetative survival in this group was also rare but is increasing due to more frequent treatment of cardio-respiratory arrest by modern emergency techniques of resuscitation. Carbon dioxide retention increases severe cerebral edema, to which the young are prone.

Post-pubertal patients recover more slowly and more serious personality disorders can persist for many years and may never resolve satisfactorily. Over the age of twenty years, coma or post-traumatic amnesia of one week or more may be followed by vegatative survival or profound disability which I find to be commonly associated with severe bilateral hemisphere involvement.

Many varieties of neurological dysfunction can occur but it is interesting to note that extrapyramidal dysfunction which results from acceleration concussion tends to be choreoathetoid in the first decade of life. In the second decade, as in Wilson's Disease, it may be characterized by the mask-like facies, speech impairment, rigidity of the cogwheel or lead pipe type and the coarse compound tremor and "pin rolling" of the full blown Parkinson's Disease associated with adults. These clinical observations, range from infancy to adult life and delineate the steady diminution in ability to recover motor, intellectual and behavioral abilities with more persistent undesirable behavioral reactions. All are associated with increasing lack of resilience to insults involving both hemispheres, directly attributable to age. The evidence suggests to me that aging of the brain begins not later than the first half of the second decade.

In a brain of relative maturity, as in a child of ten years, sudden trauma and slow recovery from prolonged acceleration concussion coma is associated commonly with progressive relearning of lost skills and follows Jacksonian-like levels of increasingly complex function in which motor, intellectual, sensory and perceptual skills may be regained. The eventual level achieved is below that prior to the accident and is commonly associated with patchy variability in psychological functions although this may be subtle. Memory (Russell, 1971) and intellect are most vulnerable and at the same time most difficult to evaluate (Smith, 1961; Richardson, 1963).

Human adaptation and compensation to brain lesions acquired early in development is as complicated as permutations and possible combinations of disease, trauma and circumstances dictate. As the child develops, we identify clinically the _dominant_ picture and the subsidiary levels of dysfunction, keeping in mind that these manifestations of neural damage will frequently change as the infant and child progresses to maturity. Various broad classifications of a functional nature have been suggested in an attempt to capture the essential characteristics of lesion, versus compensation, versus maturation and perhaps even regeneration.

Teuber (1962), in categorizing the behavioral effects of brain lesions that occur early in development, suggested that three major groups of brain injured children could be identified based on limited and artificial laboratory tasks. First, those who were manifestly normal in the first months and years of life and where on experimental testing, the difference between the normal and abnormal emerges only at later ages. Second, where differences are detectable in the yound child but disappear during development. Third, where the difference in the experimental laboratory tests given is apparent at all ages. In contrast, the late Richmond Paine (1962) took the major clinical areas in which neurological disease manifested itself in childhood and proposed that equally well defined subclinical affections and dysfunction are often to be found in children who present with behavioral problems or deviations. As the demands of society increase and educational pressures mount, such children are presenting in droves and are being medicated by the ton in a haphazard fashion which leaves much to be desired scientifically. The possible long-term effects of medication on the general health and well being of the patient are still unknown. Behavior and performance is often improved.

In none of Paine's cases had the diagnosis of "neurological dysfunction" been made prior to presentation although some parents had noted that the child was clumsy. The principle neurological findings in 40 cases were as follows: mild choreoathetosis, 16; ataxia, 2; tremor of hands, 6; hyperreflexia, 4; extensor plantar responses, 5; and clumsiness in only 9. One had a previously unrecognized spastic paraparesis and only one of the 40 was essentially normal, except for behavior.

These cases fit for the most part into Teuber's first group of children who were manifestly normal in the first years of life and where their differences emerged at a later age.

It might be appropriate to remind ourselves for one moment of the brilliant work of Karl Lashley (1963) who demonstrated so clearly and elegantly, (1) the effect of brain damage on the ability to acquire habits, (2) relearning (of the image) after a cerebral insult might require many times more practice than initial learning, (3) cortical blindness produces a greater deterioration of performance than the peripheral blindness of enucleation, and (4) the animal with an intact cortex but gross disturbance of motor control (from a spinal or cerebellar lesion) can outperform the cortically injured animal with normal limb control.

Lashley's experimental observations have provided subsequent generations of clinicians and experimentalists with sound concepts that help to categorize and understand the complex relationships that may exist between performance, learning and neurological dysfunction. I am reminded of my repeated observations of a remarkably severe athetoid undergraduate of Magdalen College whose wild bicycle rides up and down the Oxford High, his flailing limbs contorted by a thousand demons, stopped the traffic and amazed all but the rider himself who sped on, busy but unconcerned.

In contrast, the persistence of a few minor neurological signs following cerebral insult in infancy still poses the question - "Are these signs truly minor and of no prognostic importance or are they the tip of the iceberg with the underlying neuropsychological problems still to be revealed?" For example, hemiparesis present for weeks or months in infancy can disappear totally within the first year. We do not know really how to interpret with any certainty the significance of the signs that are observed in the first days, weeks or months of life or the factors that determine the degree of compensation or recovery.

There is an almost infinite variety of complex insults to the developing or mature brain - each equally fascinating in its implications for exploration of the effects of development and aging on function. Acute infections such as meningitis, even when treated, may damage the brains of children and adults but the most profound effects are seen in the very yound and the old, that is to say, the developmentally immature or the developmentally aged (Nyhan and Richardson, 1963).

Meningococcal meningitis is a valuable model for several reasons. Its diagnosis and effects were readily recognized in the days of Osler and well documented in the untreated pandemics of the 19th century. The use of Flexner's serum (1913) decreased mortality from 95 to 35 per cent but still leaving many damaged survivors. Later chemotheraputic treatment for this extraordinarily sensitive and rapidly responding organism further reduced mortality and morbidity. A simple chart, made from one of the great epidemics that occurred suggests that host resistance is poorest in the young and the elder (see figure 1). This has been confirmed by Wolff (1952) who showed that brain damage and mental retardation from meningitis (meningococcal) in treated infants diminished progressively with age in the first year of life.

The enormous demand for oxygen (and glucose) as the young brain grows rapidly in a rostral direction (Himwich, 1951), the competition by the organism for glucose in the cerebrospinal fluid and presumably elsewhere in the brain (Petersdorf and Harter, 1961), the fact that the toxin produced by the organism inhibits respiration of tissue slices and the action of succinic dehydrogenase and pyruvic oxidase, makes an attractive hypothesis as to one potential mechanism of interference with neuronal respiration, resulting in cerebral edema and neuronal death. In addition, cerebral metabolic demands increase 7 per cent with each degree Fahrenheit of fever.

The remarkably rapid <u>reversal</u> of disorientation, confusion and even coma with no apparent residuum in cases treated within a few hours of the acute onset is not unlike recovery from deep levels of anaesthesia induced by inhalation anaesthesia implying a reversible situation, provided that neuronal respiration or neuroglial metabolism has not been damaged beyond repair as in the cases described by Lindenberg (1963).

Meningitis from other organisms such as the pneumococcus both in infancy and over the age of 40 years, even when treated, usually has a devastating and permanent effect on the intellect (Spink and Su, 1960). In addition, total loss of hearing following by loss of speech, a not uncommon sequel to meningitis, gives us some insight into the relationship between learning, repetition and retention in memory - also the problem of maintaining an acquired and complex skill such as speech without adequate auditory support and feedback even though language is preserved (Kinney, 1948) (Table I).

Another interesting area relative to aging has been brought out in the study of chromosomal accidents in nature such as mongolism and allied chromosomal disorders. For example, patients with mental retardation associated with Downs syndrome often develop premature senility. Classical Alzheimer degenerative changes have been described by Jervis (1970) in association with the senility of mongolism. We do not know why growth is retarded early and then later accelerated with premature development of cataracts, aging and dementia. The cause and mechanism of action of the increased DNA is not known. Erythrocytes and leucocytes appear to have a shortened half-life. Kaback and Bernstein (1970) have shown that the rate of DNA replication in fibroblast tissue cultures of G-trisomies, compared to controls, is substantially different. As Cooke (1973) has pointed out, the basic biological disturbance in these trisomic cells is unknown but may shed light both on the problem of brain differentiation and the aging process.

Recent work on another complex experiment in nature which is in part age-dependent is still in progress. The relationship of malnutrition and undernutrition to brain and intellectual development (Cravioto, 1968 a,b; 1970; Dobbing, 1968; Cheek, 1973; Monckeberg, 1970) and the related work of Altman (1971) and others on the increased rate of cell proliferation in glia, neocortex, cortex, cerebellum and corpus callosum in stimulated animals versus controls, shows physiological and behavioral evidence of adaptive superiority in the stimulated animals despite smaller brains by weight. The nutrition story at different ages is not yet complete, but some observers feel that if survival is assured, environmental stimulation may rank with protein-calorie intake in order of importance to the individual. The effects of severe malnutrition on the brains of the elderly in concentration camps appear to be less well documented.

In closing, I would like to discuss briefly some new work which may have not only clinical implications, but has already added to the existing information concerning recovery and relearning after selective cerebral insults. Clinical evidence, some of which I have mentioned today, suggests that the capacity for spontaneous recovery is inversely proportional to the age of the mammalion brain once maturity is achieved.

Earl Walker (1964), from a lifetime of clinical observations and experimentation, has repeatedly commented that rehabilitative measures should be commenced as soon as possible, once the acute phase of the lesion has stabilized regardless of the age of the patient. In a series of papers over the last four years, Schwartzman (1970, 1971, 1972) has demonstrated that young adult Rhesus (macaque) monkeys can be trained to discriminate proprioception, vibration, light touch and two point discrimination. Following removal of the classical somatosensory lemniscal cortex (areas SI and SII), there was complete loss of proprioceptive and two point discriminatory ability with minimal loss of vibration and light touch.

The animals were subjected immediately to extensive retraining and animals regained all fine sensory function (except for a slight decrease of sensitivity for proprioceptive and two point thresholds). The critical difference between this and prior work is that the retraining period was instituted immediately and systematically. Surprisingly good results were also obtained following medullary pyramidal section despite some residual weakness, slowness and selective increase in tone of forelimb flexors, hip adductors, ankle extensors and foot invertors.

Schwartzman has worked recently with children with infantile hemiplegia; for example, one child with a hemiplegia of 17 months duration, severe right sided with a palmar adducted thumb and permanently fisted, a right homonymous hemianopsia, severe spasticity and impaired light touch and pinprick. After one month of intensive retraining improvement was noted. After four months of training an excellent pincer grasp and good release had developed. Of great interest and probable significance is that the child appeared to learn by observing his own mirror movements made first by the unaffected limb and hand and then persevering in trying to reproduce them in the affected limb. At six months associated movements started to return, although spasticity, hemisensory deficit and hypereflexia remained unchanged. Similar improvement has been noted in hemiathietosis and hemiparesis. It is important to note these children were intelligent and had no clinical evidence of bilateral hemipshere involvement.

In this discussion I have mentioned but a few of the experiments in nature by which we are surrounded and which afford us opportunity to study the complex effects of age on the brain's responses. Samuel Butler said, ..."one of the arts of living consists in the ability to come to adequate conclusions from inadequate evidence". It is perhaps fortunate that we do not always have to live by the hypotheses we make until we have adequate evidence to substantiate or refute them.

REFERENCES

Altman, J. (1971). In "Brain Development and Behavior" (M.B. Sterman, J. McGinty and M. Adinolfi, eds.), Academic Press, New York.

André-Thomas, Chesni, Y. and Saint-Anne Dargassies, S. (1960). In "The Neurological Examination of the Infant" (R.C. MacKeith, P.E. Polani and E. Clayton-Jones, eds.), p. 23, National Spastics Society, London.

Birch, H.G. (1964). "Brain Damage in Children." Williams and Wilkins, Baltimore.

Black, P. (1973). Personal communication.

Blackwood, W., Meyer, A., Norman, R. and McMenemey, W.H. (1963). "Greenfield's Neuropathology." Williams and Wilkins, Baltimore.

Brierley, J.B. (1971). In "Brain Hypoxia" (J.B. Brierley and B.S. Meldrum, eds.), p. 306, The Lavenham Press, Suffolk.

Cheek, D.B. (1973). In "Brain and Intelligence. The Ecology of Child Development" (F. Richardson, ed.), National Educational Press, Hyattsville, Maryland.

Cooke, R.E. (1973). In "Brain and Intelligence. The Ecology of Child Development" (F. Richardson, ed.), pp. 315-331, National Educational Press, Hyattsville, Maryland.

Cravioto, J. (1968a). In "Malnutrition, Learning and Behavior" (S. Scrimshaw and J.E. Gordon, eds.), pp.252-268, M.I.T. Press, Cambridge.
Cravioto, J. (1968b). In "Expanding Concepts in Mental Retardation" (G.A. Jervis, ed.), pp. 63-76, Thomas, Springfield, Illinois.
Denny-Brown, D. (1966). "The Cerebral Control of Movement". Thomas, Springfield, Illinois.
Denny-Brown, D. and Russell, W.R. (1941). Brain 64, 93.
Dobbing, J. (1968). In "Expanding Concepts in Mental Retardation" (A. Jervis, ed.), pp. 77-85, Thomas, Springfield, Illinois.
Eccles, J.C. (1968). In "Growth of the Nervous System" (G.E.W. Wolstenholme and M. O'Connor, eds.), J & A Churchill Ltd., London.
Eccles, J.C. (1973). J. Physiol. 229, 1.
Flatten, H. (1906). Klin. Jahrb. XV, 211.
Flexner, S. (1913). J. Exptl. Med. 17, 553.
Ford, F. (1960). Personal communication.
Himwich, H. (1951). "Brain Metabolism and Cerebral Disorders." Williams and Wilkins, Baltimore.
Holburn, A.H.S. (1945). Brit. Med. Bull. 3, 147.
Holmes, Sir Gordon (1968). "Introduction to Clinical Neurology." Livingston, London.
Jervis, G.A. (1970). Ann. N.Y. Acad. Sci. 171, 559.
Johnson, R. (1972). New Eng. J. Med. 287, 599.
Kaback, M.M. and Bernstein, L.H. (1970). Ann. N.Y. Acad. Sci. 171, 526.
Kinney, C. (1948). Arch Otolaryngol. 47, 303.
Környey, S. (1963). In "Selective Vulnerability of the Brain in Hypoxaemia" (J.P. Schade and W.H. McMenemey, eds.), pp. 165-176, Davis, Philadelphia.
Lashley, K.S. (1963). "Brain Mechanisms and Intelligence." Dover Publications, New York.
Lindenberg, R. (1963). In "Selective Vulnerability of the Brain in Hypoxaemia" (J.P. Schade and W.H. McMenemey, eds.), pp. 211-226, Davis, Philadelphia.
Malamud, N. (1963). In "Selective Vulnerability of the Brain in Hypoxaemia" (J.P. Schade and W.H. McMenemey, eds.), pp. 211-226, Davis, Philadelphia.
Monckeberg, F.B. (1973). In "Brain and Intelligence. The Ecology of Child Development" (F. Richardson, ed.), pp. 207-229, National Educational Press, Hyattsville, Maryland.

Nyhan, W.L. and Richardson, F. (1963). Ann. Review Med. 14, 243.
Paine, R. (1962). Dev. Med. Child. Neurol. 4, 21.
Peiper, A. (1961). "Cerebral Function in Infancy and Childhood." Consultants Bureau, New York, 1963.
Petersdorf, R.G. and Harter, D.H. (1961). Arch. Neurol. 4, 21.
Prechtl, H. and Beintena, D. (1964). "The Neurological Examination of the Full-Term Newborn Infant." The Spastics Society Medical Education and Information Unit and William Heinemann Medical Books, London.
Pudenz, R.H. and Shelden, C.H. (1946). J. Neurosurg. 3,487.
Richardson, F. (1963). Dev. Med. Child. Neurol. 5, 471.
Richardson, F. (1965). Unpublished observations.
Richardson, F. (1968). In "Physical Trauma as an Etiological Agent in Mental Retardation", U.S. Dept. of Health, Education and Welfare, Washington, D.C. 20402.
Russell, W.R. (1971). "The Traumatic Amnesias." Oxford University Press, London.
Schwartzman, R.J. (1970). Arch.Neurol. 23, 419.
Schwartzman, R.J. (1971). Exptl. Neurol. 33, 147.
Schwartzman, R.J. (1972). Arch.Neurol. 27, 340.
Sherrington, C. (1961). "The Integrative Action of the Nervous System." Yale University Press, New Haven.
Shiraki, H. (1968). In "Wilson's Disease" (D. Bergesma, ed.), The National Foundation, New York.
Smith, A. (1961). Dis. Nerv. Syst. 22, 69.
Spink, W. and Su. C. (1960). J. Am. Med. Assoc. 173, 1545.
Teuber, H.L. and Rudel, R.G. (1962). Dev. Med. Child. Neurol. 4, 3.
Walker, A.E. (1964). Personal communication.
Windle, F. (1958). In "Neurological and Psychological Deficits of Asphyxia Neonatorum" (W.F. Windle, ed.), Thomas, Springfield, Illinois.
Wolff, O.H. (1952). Arch. Dis. Child. 27, 302.

TABLE I

Deafness From Meningitis

Age at Onset in Years	Words	Voice Change	Total Loss of Speech
Under 1-1/2	10	At once	At once
2	50	At once	8 weeks
3	Normal for age	3 weeks	6 weeks
4	Normal for age	8 weeks	6 months
6	Normal for age	3 months	2 years
10	Normal for age	6 months	18 months
18	Normal for age	1 year	3 years
19	Normal for age	1 year	Not lost

N.B. With increasing age, memory for voice quality and speech is retained for longer periods following the acute insult. (Adapted from Kinney, C., Arch. Otolaryngol. 47: 303, 1948.)

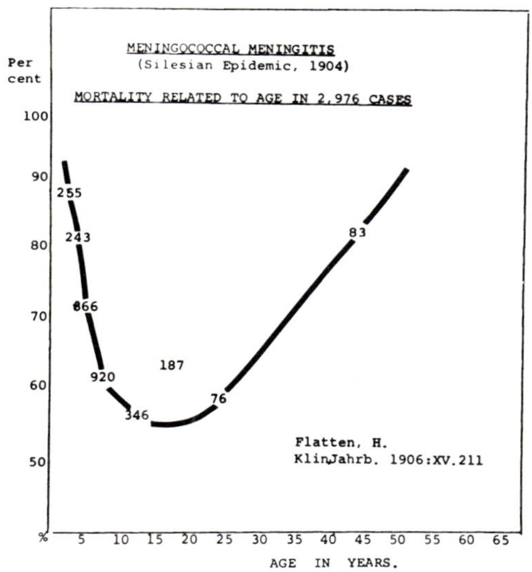

Fig. 1 In the Silesian pandemic of 1904, 2,976 patients of all ages died. (Mortality rates usually exceeded ninety percent.) The percentage mortality related to the different age groups shows that maximum vulnerability occurred in the first and fourth decade onwards. (Adapted from Flatten, H., Klin, Jarhb. 1906: XV, 211.)

NEUROCHEMICAL PATTERNS IN THE DEVELOPING AND AGING BRAIN

Williamina A. Himwich

Nebraska Psychiatric Institute
602 South 44th Avenue
Omaha, Nebraska 68105

In the last twenty years the interest in developmental biology, especially as it applies to the developing brain, has grown by leaps and bounds. It is, however, I think, an unfortunate commentary on much of the neurochemical data that, while it is of itself excellent, it has not been planned to fit into any overall scheme of elucidating our knowledge of brain development. Many theses have been and are being planned in departments of biochemistry to explain a neurochemical problem. Biochemists inevitably look upon the brain as another biochemical milieu and are not interested in the functional aspects of biochemical development. Development, almost by coincidence, is associated with the problem. The reasons for this approach of course are obvious, but I am hoping that as the new crop of students prepare their doctoral theses in neurochemistry, they will be encouraged to have a broader viewpoint of the functional importance of neurochemistry.

To a large extent, the correlation between behavior and neurochemistry, even in the developing animal, has been disappointing. This lack is not due to the fact that no such correlation exists, but simply because we, as neurochemists, have not been able to look at the right places in the brain. We have been comparing, and are still comparing chemical constituents present in whole brain or in brain areas and attempting to relate these changes to behavior. Many of these substances are of importance at the synapses (for example, GABA) and small changes in concentration at these sites can be expected to produce changes in function or behavior. In determining overall concentrations in a group of cells representing either whole brain or anatomically discreet areas of the brain, such significant changes are lost. The difficulty in connecting function with neurochemistry is well illustrated in the drug field, where marked changes are frequently seen in substances considered to be neurotransmitters without a measurable change in function. We are still in a very early state of attempting to relate these two parameters. This problem is of importance not only in development, but is of even more urgency in the aged animal.

As neurochemists we have a number of acute technical needs before we can do a better job. One is the ability to prepare reproducible fractions of neurons, of glia, of synaptosomes, and of other cell fragments. When I say reproducible, I am not referring to relatively pure preparations which now can be obtained rather easily under carefully controlled conditions, but to preparations which from one day to the next are a reasonable facsimile of each other. Such preparations are needed if we wish to study animals over an age span and we do not yet have that ability (Lempkey-Johnston and Dekirmenjian, 1970).

Another problem that faces us is the fact that animals are raised under a wide variety of conditions which contribute, in essentially unknown quantities, to the variability of the data. We now know that many things such as handling, time of killing, period of light and dark, etc., can influence neurochemistry, especially in the young animal. We also see papers from innumerable laboratories studying approximately the same conditions, but going about it in an entirely different fashion. These papers are often not comparable and, although of value in themselves, we cannot use them for comparative data. Moreover, studies done on rats often cannot be translated into studies on cats and, still more important, cannot be extrapolated to studies on man. It seems to me that, certainly in the field of development and of aging, there can be no question that our interests lie fundamentally in understanding human brain development and how the brain ages. Therefore, we are deluding ourselves and ignoring the main problem, if our experimental designs do not permit extrapolation of our data to man.

We have begun to seek a solution to this quandary in developing brain studies. Throughout the last 20 years, the research group associated with me has studied various species of animals using, as nearly as possible, the same biochemical techniques, even though this, at times, has meant that we were using techniques in 1970 which were more appropriate to the early 1960's. We have deliberately pursued this course in order to obtain strictly comparable data across species. These data we are now analyzing to see the possibilities of judging rates of development at various times during pre- and postnatal life and of determining whether there are times in the life of each of the species when the rate of brain development or of acquisition of any given substance important to cerebral metabolism is the same as that in another species and, of course, in man. The studies of Dobbing (1970) and his analyses of data have moved in somewhat the same direction (Fig. 1).

For our work, we have divided the period from conception to the attainment of a mature brain weight into 20 equal periods for all species. This adjustment of chronological time has made it possible for us to draw on a single graph the rate of accumulation of any given brain constituent for several species. These lines then give a family of curves which can be compared. For example, brain weight is the parameter in which data on the greatest number of species are available. The growth of the brain can be expressed as the percent of adult weight reached at any given period of time. These curves are similar (Fig. 2). However, they obviously have different slopes at different times. Is it possible that they have the same slope at some point in developmental time? In order to determine this we simply eliminated the horizontal axis and moved the curves together until there were sections in which the lines were parallel (Fig. 3). These zones of intersection or parallelism can then be translated back into ages and we obtain a table of age equivalents (Table 1) which can be used to determine when a cat, for example, might be studied in order to produce data which could give some estimates of what is happening in human brain at specified time. Such curves, perhaps, can give us a starting point. And, as more data are accumulated, more comparisons can be made, more curves can be drawn, and more estimations of age equivalents can be made. It would be very helpful if we could use brain weight as the basis of age equivalents for all brain constituents. Let me show you, however, what happens with a brain region, such as the hippocampus, when we attempt to compare the age equivalents in changes of glutamic acid concentration (Fig. 4). In this case, there is only a short period of coincidence of curves for the three species that have been studied. We cannot be sure what the situation would be in man since no data are available. Obviously, more data for all species and for all ages are necessary before we can refine this technique.

As a background for a discussion of aging, I would like to summarize the changes which occur with maturation in the mammalian brain irrespective of the species. If we use data from human brain, we can see a gradual increase in brain weight which then plateaus (Fig. 5). There is a fall in moisture as the brain acquires myelin and as protein is deposited with a concomitant increase in dry material. Simultaneously, lipids increase principally as myelination progresses. A decrease in DNA and RNA content per unit volume accompanies maturation, since the cells become more widely spread by the development of the neuropil. Therefore, as the brain matures, any given volume of tissue contains less of those substances which are peculiar to the cell body. In general, the enzymatic patterns follow much the same sort of development. In other words, there are marked increases of most constituents as the brain is maturing with a flattening of the curves at maturity.

Such an overall picture as I have described above, of course, says nothing of what is happening in the brain parts. We must remember, that in some animals, the hippocampus, for example, is nearly mature at birth, at least as far as the synaptic organization is concerned (Purpura _et al_., 1964). The pons-medulla is also mature. In general, we can speak of a caudal-rostral development whereby the most caudal structures mature the earliest and the most rostral the latest. The hippocampus is an exception to this, and I suspect that there are other exceptions, if we looked for them. For instance, the visual tract is functional electrophysiologically, at least to electrical stimulation of the optic nerve, long before the retina has matured (Hunt and Goldring, 1951). Anokhin (1964) has pointed out that there are differences, even in given nuclei in the brain in the rate in which neurons develop. Their prime example has been the development of neurons in the facial nucleus which control the muscles necessary for sucking. It is simplistic to attempt to consider only the caudal to rostral development. On the other hand, as with many other simple explanations, this one has contributed a great deal to our understanding and knowledge of the overall development of the brain (Himwich, 1951).

The above picture, in its overall dimensions, shows what happens in the brain as the neural streak develops to maturity. What kinds of changes occur after the brain is mature? Is it possible to give as general a picture for aging in all species as we can for development? If we start with man as the focal point of our interest, changes in other species must be related to changes in human brain, so that we can decide how comparable the species are. Of necessity then, we should consider first the only comprehensive study done on aging man. Bürger (1957) in East Germany followed cases at autopsy and determined constituents of brain such as moisture, dry weight, total lipids, protein, etc. In man there appeared to be a definite pattern of aging in which after the sixth decade of life, the brain became smaller and contained more water (Fig. 6). At the same time, protein and lipid were decreasing. If we are to accept this work of Bürger (which we are forced to do since it is all we have), then we should consider what species of animals gives us the best approximation of conditions as they occur in the senile human brain. It has been known since the time of Donaldson (1924) that the rat brain continues to grow, although at a very slow rate, as long as the animal lives. The same appears true for all rodents, but not for dogs and cats (Table 2). We have investigated over many years the brains of aged animals of several species as they became available. From these data on water content it is not possible to be sure whether or not rabbit brain begins to accumulate water at old age (Table 3). The brains from old dogs and cats seem more moist than those in younger animals, although the data are still too few for us to draw any firm quantitative conclusions.

I would like now to turn to the work that Mr. Davis and I have just completed on brains of rhesus monkeys ranging from 3 to 16 years of age. We secured these animals through the kindness of Dr. J. Mark Ordy of Northern University of Illinois at DeKalb. These animals were raised at the Cleveland Zoo and used by Dr. Ordy as breeding stock. In sampling brains from these animals, we were faced with the problem of whether we should attempt to study whole brain or brain parts. Since we have come, more and more, to the conclusion that the parts of the brain will eventually yield more information than the whole brain *per se*, we decided to use these animals only for a study of brain parts. With the small number of animals available, only tentative conclusions can be drawn at this time. For DNA and RNA content of most brain parts, the maximum content occurred either at 3 to 4 years, but in the occipital, motor and parietal cortices, at 8 to 10 years (Fig. 7 and 8). After that time, there appeared to be a decrease in DNA, noticeable especially in the parietal and the temporal cortices. In the case of RNA, the fall is much more striking (Fig. 9 and 10) suggesting that, although the DNA remains relatively intact, its ability to manufacture and utilize RNA decreases as the animal ages. Protein content, in general, shows shifts with age, especially in certain cortical areas (Fig. 11). In some parts, however, the RNA present is sufficient to maintain the necessary protein synthesis. Except for the cerebellum and the caudate nucleus, the other brain parts have a slight decrease in DNA at 15 to 16 years of age (Fig. 8). The decrease is greater in RNA than DNA in these parts, as it was in the cortical areas, and there is some evidence of a decrease in protein which is probably not significant (Fig. 12). In the same parts also, acetylcholinesterase showed a tendency to decrease at that age with the greatest fall occurring in the parietal cortex and in the cervical spinal cord. Acetylcholinesterase decreased in the cerebellum and had a tendency to fall in all parts except the superior colliculi. In the thalamus, almost 50% is lost by age 15-16 years. In interpreting these data, the limited number of animals studied at each of the various ages must be considered. The possibility that some of the animals (possibly the oldest) had some brain pathology should not be underestimated. We cannot guess at the nature of the pathology, but since many viral diseases and parasitic infections result in damage to the brain (Turbes, personal communication), it is possible that these animals suffered such damage.

Unfortunately, the monkey brain samples were not large enough to allow us to assay free amino acids on this particular group of animals. For the study of what happens to the free amino acid content, we must turn to other species. Early work from our laboratory seemed to show that for the whole rat brain there was a marked decrease in glutamic acid and glutamine as the animal aged (Fig.13). Recently, data on the hamster have been collected over a period of two years involving 12 animals in each age group. In these animals, there was a marked decrease in glutamic acid content, as well as a fall in GABA and in aspartic acid content. At the same time, there was very little change in protein content of the whole brain. The moisture content of the hamster brain, likewise changed very little during the period from two months to two years (Fig. 14).

One area that has been neglected in studies of the aging brain is that of overall cerebral metabolic rate (CMR). In man, "normal" subjects 56-79 years of age (Scheinberg *et al*., 1953) and those with senile dementia (Freyhan *et al*., 1951) show a marked decrease in CMR. In aged dogs, we have found a decrease in *in vitro* oxygen consumption even in the medulla (Himwich and Himwich,1959). Such a decrease in metabolic activity may be a more sensitive indicator of behavioral changes in the aged animal than neurochemical changes. The latter may be secondary to the changes in nutrition of the cells.

Research on aged animals is expensive largely because of the cost of maintaining the animal until they reach a "ripe old age". However, such research is desperately needed if we are to understand the process of aging as it affects the brain.

ACKNOWLEDGEMENT

In concluding, I would like to thank my many colleagues, especially Dr. H. C. Agrawal, Dr. Anant Dravid, J. M. Davis, and David Callison as well as the skillful technicians who assisted in the acquisition of the data.

REFERENCES

Anokhin, P.K. (1964). *In* "The Developing Brain" (W.A. Himwich and H.W. Himwich, eds.), *Prog. Brain Res.* *4*, 55, Elsevier, Amsterdam.

Bürger, M. (1957). *Abhandl. säcks. Akad. Wies, Leipwig. Math. - naturw. Kl.* *45*, 1.

Dobbing, J. (1970). In "Developmental Neurobiology" (W.A. Himwich, ed.), pp. 241-261, Charles C. Thomas, Springfield, Illinois.

Donaldson, H.H. (1924). In "The Rat", Memoirs of the Wistar Institute of Anatomy and Biology, No. 6, Philadelphia.

Freyhan, F.A., Woodford, R.B. and Kety, S.S. (1951). J. Nervous Mental Disease 113, 449.

Himwich, H.E. (1951). "Brain Metabolism and Cerebral Disorders." Chapter 7, Williams and Wilkins, Baltimore.

Himwich, W.A. (1971). In "The Biopsychology of Development" (E. Tobach, L.R. Aronson and E. Shaw, eds.), pp. 173-194, Academic Press, New York.

Himwich, W.A. and Himwich, H.E. (1959). In "Handbook of Aging and the Individual" (J.E. Birren, ed.), pp. 187-215, University of Chicago Press, Chicago.

Hunt, W.E. and Goldring, S. (1951). Electroencephalog. Clin. Neurophysiol. 3, 465.

Lempkey-Johnston, N. and Dekirmenjian, H. (1970). Exp. Brain Res. 11, 392.

Purpura, D.P., Shofer, R.J., Housepian, E.M. and Noback, C.R. (1964). In "Growth and Maturation of the Brain" (D.P. Purpura and J.P. Schadé, eds.), Prog. Brain Res. 4, 187, Elsevier, Amsterdam.

Scheinberg, P., Blackburn, I., Rich, M. and Saslaw, M. (1953). Arch. Neurol. 70, 77.

TABLE 1
AGE EQUIVALENTS % ADULT LEVELS
(Total Brain Weight)

	START INTERSECTION	END INTERSECTION
HUMAN	15.5 Mos. After Birth	20 Mos. After Birth
RAT	13 Days After Birth	17.5 Days After Birth
HUMAN	6.3 Mos. Fetal	1 Mo. After Birth
MONKEY	75 Days Fetal	110 Days Fetal
HUMAN	7 Mos. Fetal	5 Mos. After Birth
CAT	59 Days Fetal	15 Days After Birth
RAT	9 Days After Birth	20 Days After Birth
RABBIT	9.5 Days After Birth	18 Days After Birth
RAT	Birth	26.5 Days After Birth
HAMSTER	3.3 Days After Birth	17.4 Days After Birth

TABLE 2
CHANGES IN BRAIN WEIGHT WITH AGING
(grams)

SPECIES	MATURE ADULT	AGED	YEARS TAKEN AS AGED	% DIFFERENCE FROM ADULT
MAN	1380	1240	70+	- 10.1
RHESUS MONKEY	82.5	------	---	-----
DOG	71.8	62.3	15	- 13.2
CAT	25.6	24.3	10+	- 5.1
GUINEA PIG	4.22	3.87	5+	- 8.3
RABBIT	8.3	9.8	5+	+ 14.9
RAT	1.82	1.85	2+	+ 1.6
HAMSTER	1.08	1.24	2+	+ 12.9
MOUSE	0.44	0.46	2+	+ 4.3

TABLE 3

WATER CONTENT IN AGED MAMMALIAN BRAIN
(Percent of whole brain)

	60-70 Days	3.5 Months	1 Year	2 Years	3 Years	4 Years	6 Years	8 Years
GUINEA PIG	80.4	78.9	77.1	79.8	78.7	77.9	80.1	----
MOUSE	80.7	80.5	80.3	76.7	----	----	----	----
HAMSTER	78.2	78.3	79.6	77.8	----	----	----	----
RABBIT	79.7	79.9	80.C	78.5	77.9	79.3	76.4	75.5

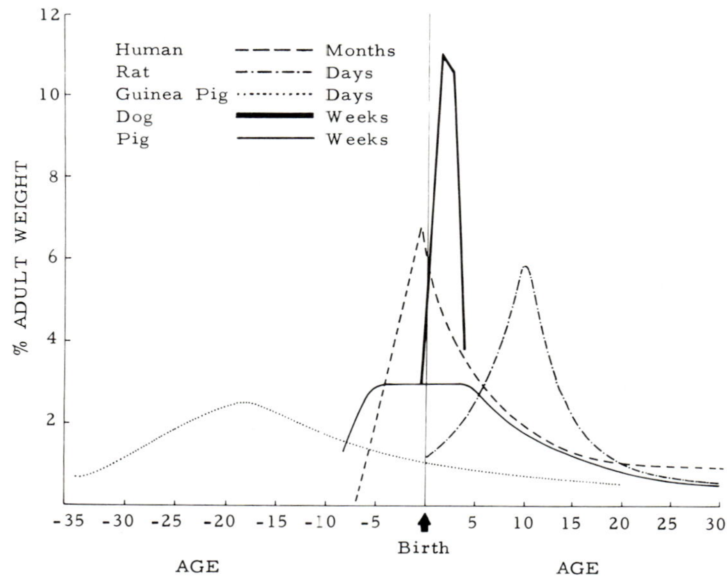

Fig. 1 Rates of brain growth in different species. Taken from Dobbing (1970).

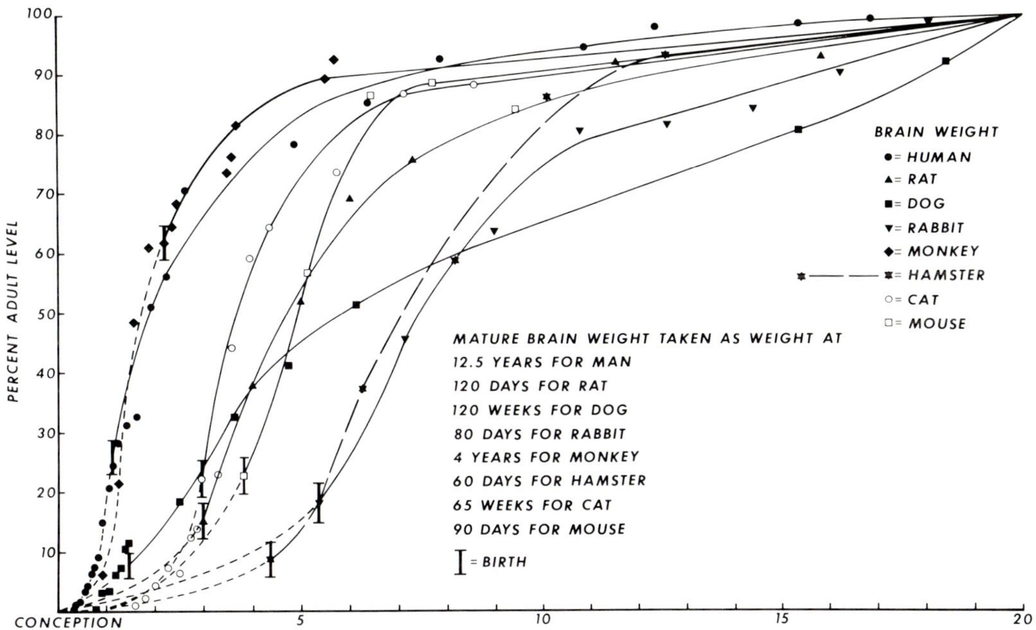

Fig. 2 Brain growth in various species. Ordinate: percent of adult level, absicca: period from conception to mature weight divided into twenty equal periods.

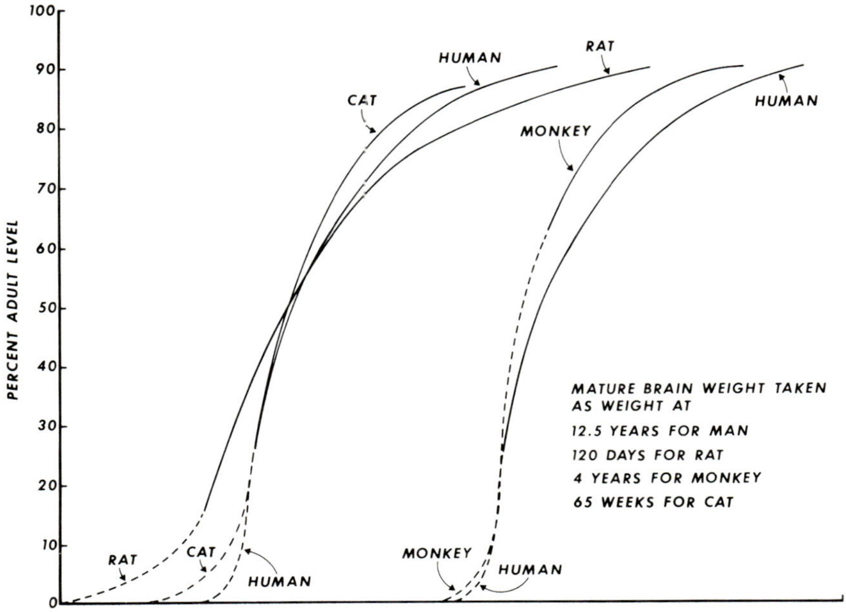

Fig. 3 Intersections of brain growth curves for various species. See Table 1 of ages.

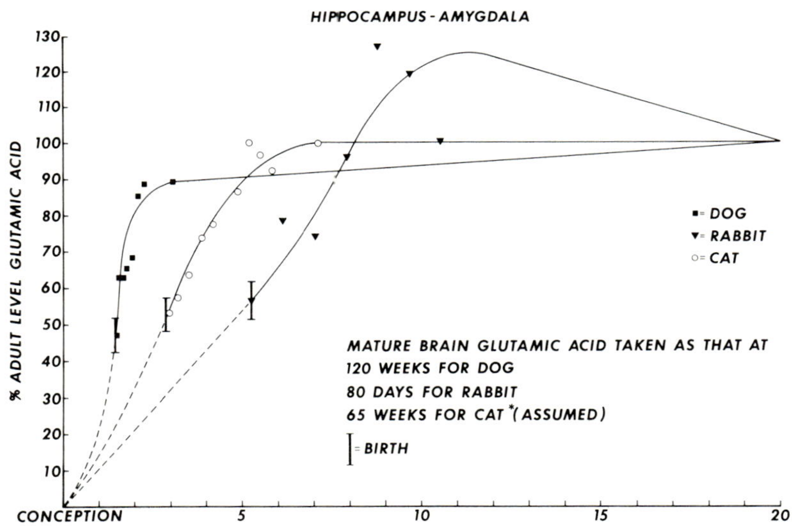

Fig. 4 Accumulation of glutamic acid in hippocampus-amygdala of various species. Absissa: period from conception to adult level divided into twenty periods.

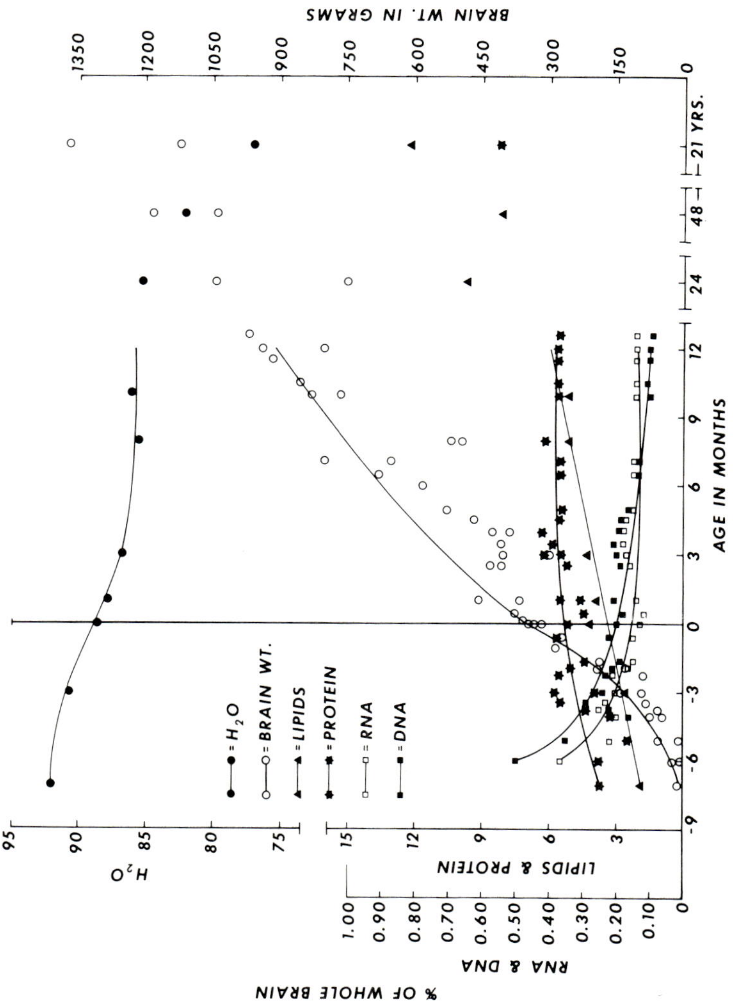

Fig. 5 Development of human brain. Taken from Himwich (1971).

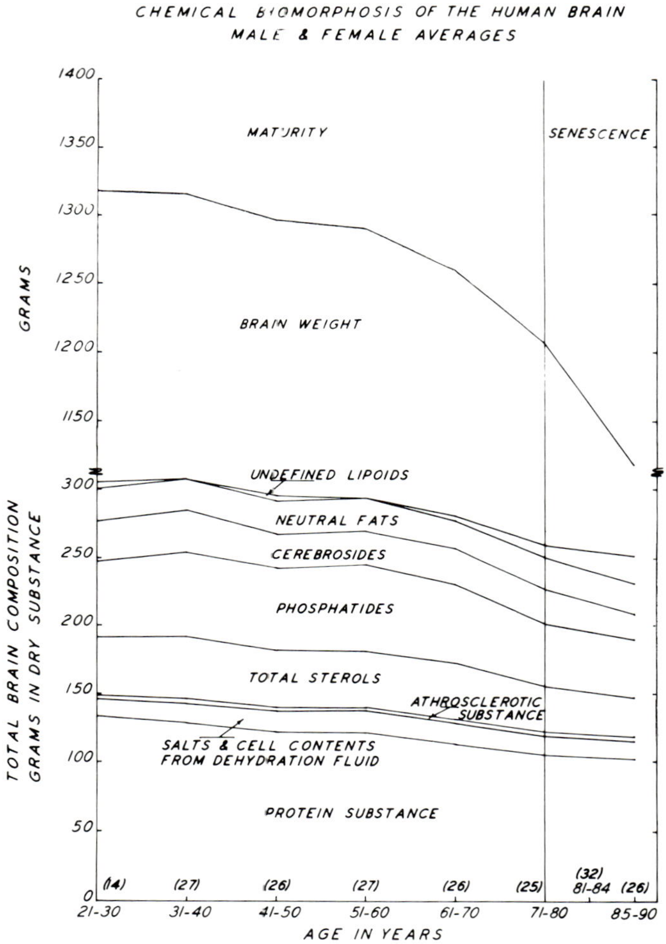

Fig. 6 Taken from Bürger (1957).

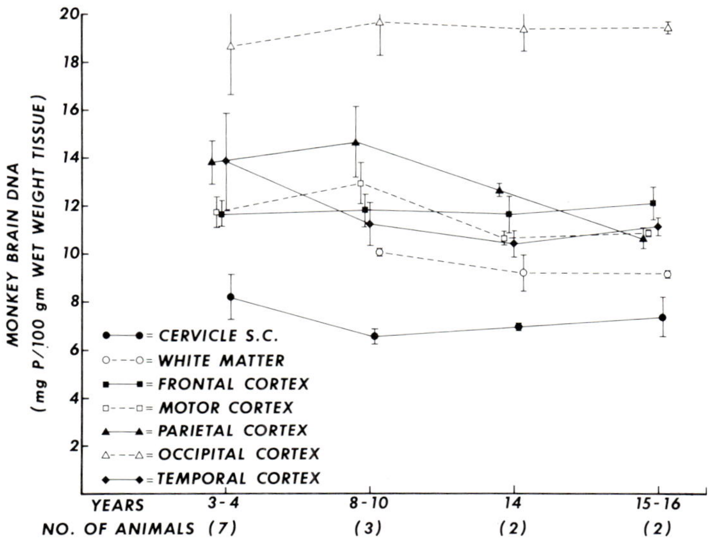

Fig. 7 DNA in monkey brain parts at various ages.

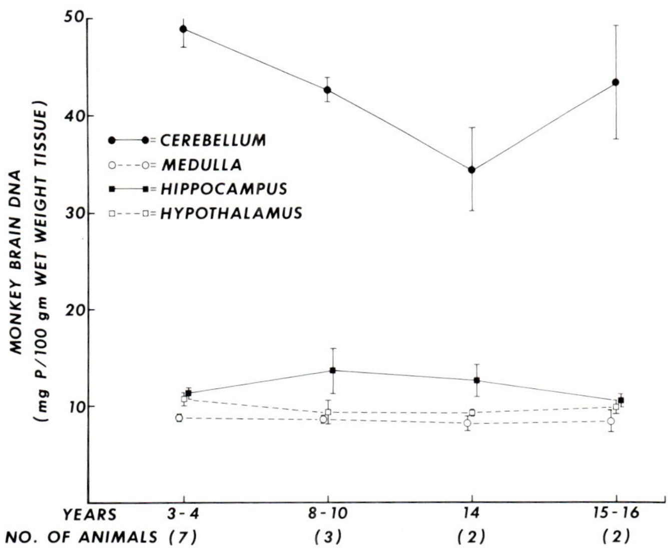

Fig. 8 DNA in monkey brain parts at various ages.

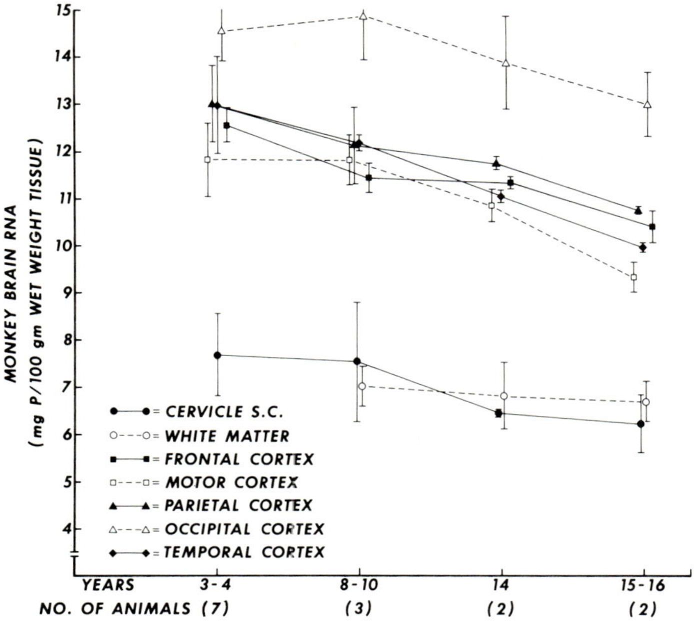

Fig. 9 RNA in monkey brain at various ages.

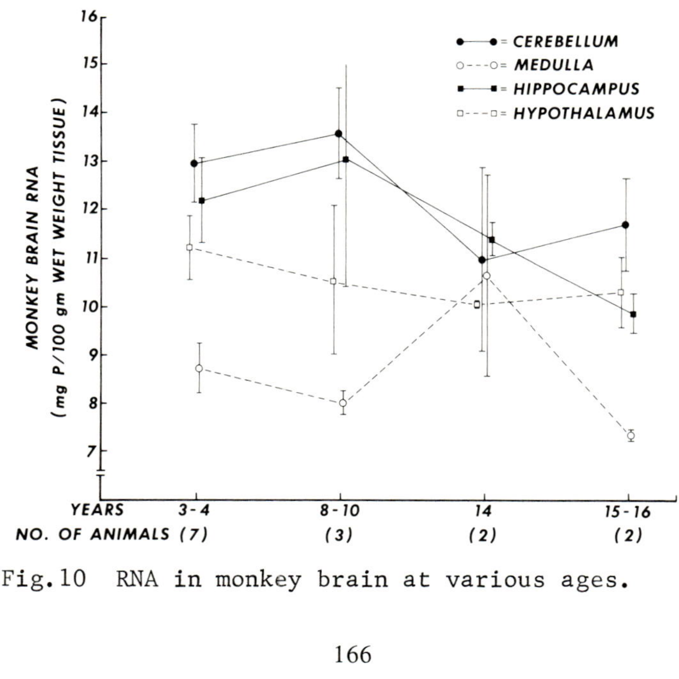

Fig.10 RNA in monkey brain at various ages.

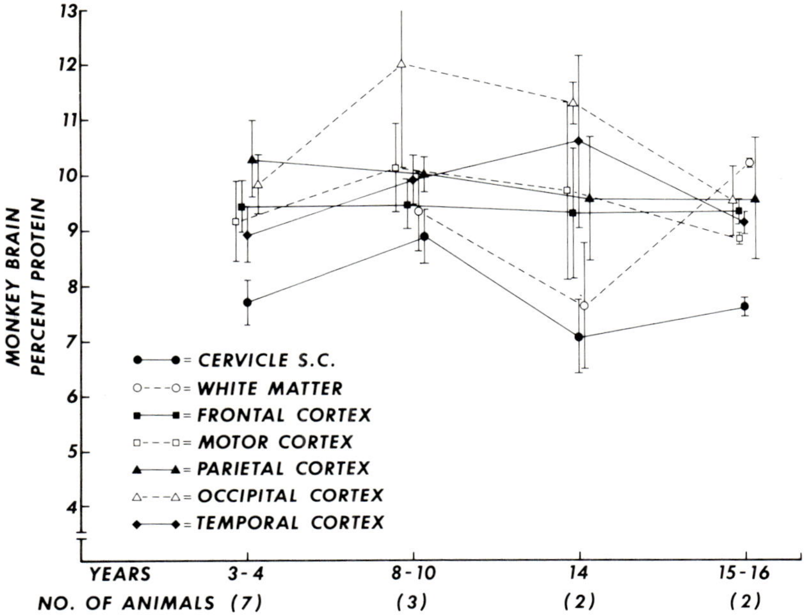

Fig.11 Percent protein in monkey brain at various ages.

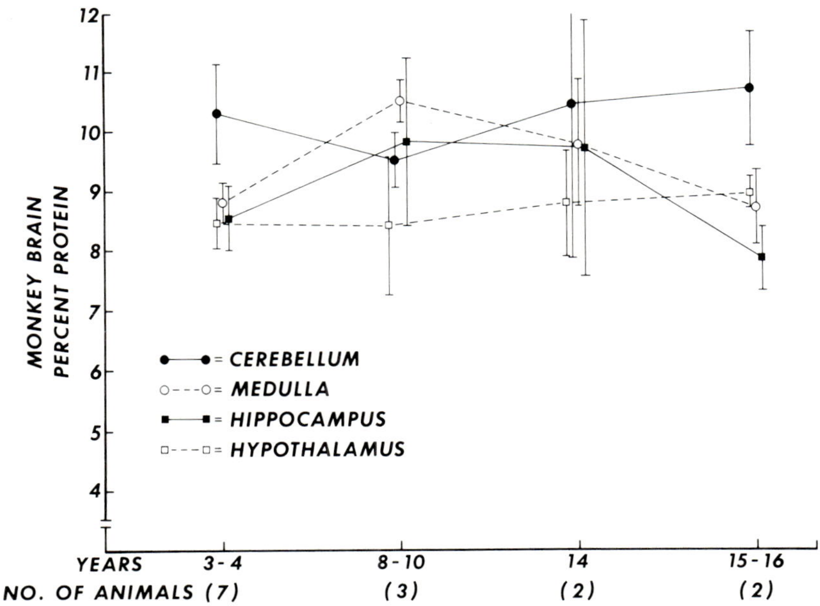

Fig.12 Percent protein in monkey brain at various ages.

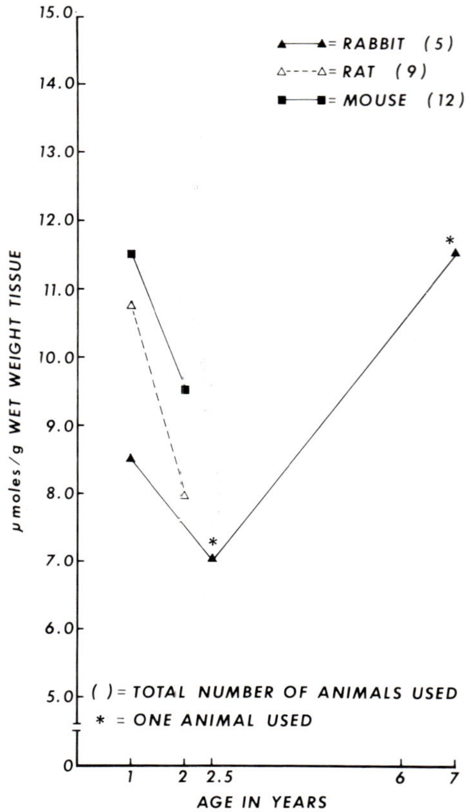

Fig.13 Glutamic acid content in aging mammalian brain.

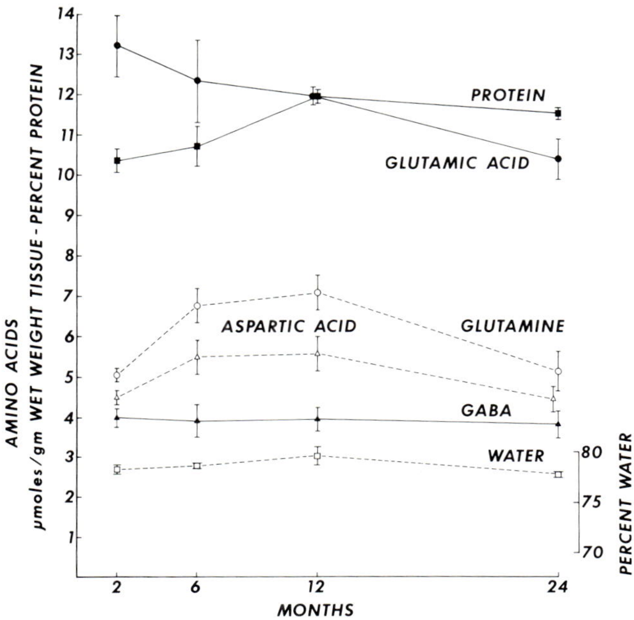

Fig.14 Neurochemical effects of aging in hamster whole brain.

MECHANISMS OF ENZYMATIC DIFFERENTIATION IN THE BRAIN AND IN CULTURED CELLS

Jean de Vellis

Laboratory of Nuclear Medicine and Radiation Biology
Department of Anatomy and Mental Retardation Center
University of California School of Medicine
Los Angeles, California 90024

Introduction

The enzyme profile of a tissue determines its functional potential. Specific changes in enzyme levels, rather than changes in catalytic functions of a fixed amount of enzyme, seem to be the general rule during development (de Vellis, 1970). Changes in enzyme activities resulting from selective gene activation or repression is thought to be the primary mechanism of cell differentiation. It is also known that changes in the proportion of various enzymes occur in aging, and it has been suggested that the event is genetic and of a quasi-differentiated nature. On the other hand, Orgel (1963) has proposed that aging results from the alteration of enzyme properties through an accumulation of errors in protein synthesis. In support of this hypothesis Holliday and Tarrant (1972) have recently reported that enzymes in aging human fibroblasts have increased heat lability.

To resolve the process of differentiation or aging, it appears easiest to focus on individual key enzymes for which stimuli regulating their selective synthesis are known. In our laboratory we have found that brain glycerophosphate dehydrogenase (GPDH) is regulated by cortisol and that lactate dehydrogenase (LDH) is controlled by catecholamines and cyclic AMP. Our present report deals with the regulation of the level of these two enzymes in the developing and adult brain and in cultured brain cells.

In the developing rat brain, most enzymes (e.g., malate dehydrogenase; see fig. 1) increase two- to threefold during the first three postnatal weeks, the critical period of Flexner (de Vellis and Clemente, 1970). On the other hand, a few enzymes, such as isocitrate dehydrogenase (fig. 1), decrease in activity. Following this critical period, there is a second period of enzyme development which lasts until 40 days of age, during which GPDH (fig.1), S-100 protein, a brain specific protein (Herschman _et al._, 1971), and carbonic anhydrase (Millichop, 1957) are induced. This second period of postnatal enzyme development follows glial proliferation which suggests that these three proteins may originate from glial cells. Carbonic anhydrase is present in glial cells of Deiter's nucleus but not in neurons (Giacobini, 1964). S-100 protein is also thought to be of glial cell origin because its concentration in the optic nerve rises during degeneration of axons of the optic nerve (Perez _et al._, 1970) and it is characteristically high in glial tumors and glial cell lines (Benda _et al._, 1968). Similarly GPDH concentration increases during degeneration of the optic nerve (McCaman and Robins, 1959) and is inducible in the same cell line as S-100 protein (de Vellis and Inglish, 1969). However, these three proteins appear to be under separate control. Unlike GPDH, S-100 (Herschman _et al._, 1971) and carbonic anhydrase (de Vellis, unpublished data) are not regulated by pituitary hormones or the glands regulated by them in developing or adult rat brains. Even though GPDH exists at various levels in most tissues, its induction by cortisol and its developmental profile is specific to brain tissue. For example, GPDH developes prenatally in the liver (Burch _et al._, 1963) and postnatally in the brain as we mentioned earlier.

Wistar rats were raised in our vivarium. All injections were performed subcutaneously in the nape of the neck.

RGC_6 cells, rat glial tumor cells, C_6 strain (Benda _et al._, 1968) are grown as monolayers in T-30 or T-250 F Falcon plastic flasks. The culture medium is 3 ml for T-30 flasks and 10 ml for T-250 flasks of Ham's F-10 (GIBCO) containing 10% virus-screened fetal calf serum (Reheis) without antibiotics. All cultures are kept at 37° C in incubators gassed with a 5% CO_2, 95% air mixture. All clones obtained from the C_6 strain are diploid and their karyotypes are undistinguishable from that of normal rat cells. Cultures were free from mycoplasma. Virus C particles have not been seen in electron micrographs (de Vellis *et al.*, 1971a). Clones are kept at a low passage number by freezing stock of cells in liquid nitrogen. Continuing stocks are passed every 6 to 8 months.

Brains were dissected out, tissues homogenized and enzymes assayed as previously described (de Vellis *et al.*, 1967; de Vellis and Inglish, 1968). Cell cultures were harvested in 0.1 M phosphate buffer adjusted to pH 7.3 and homogenized. One unit of enzyme is defined as that amount which will catalyze the transformation of 1 nanomole of substrate/min. at 30° C. Specific activity is expressed as units of enzymes/mg of (total tissue) protein.

Induction of Glycerophosphate Dehydrogenase by Cortisol in the Rat Brain

Glycerophosphate dehydrogenase (E.C.1.1.1.8) is a soluble cytoplasmic enzyme which is NAD^+-dependent. GPDH catalyzes the conversion of dihydroxyacetone phosphate to glycerophosphate. The reaction is reversible, but its equilibrium favors glycerophosphate. Mitochondrial glycerophosphate dehydrogenase, a very different protein, is a flavoprotein which converts glycerophosphate to dihydroxyacetone phosphate. This reaction is irreversible and uses oxygen. These two enzymes can work together to form the glycerophosphate cycle which net result is to generate NAD^+ from NADH. NAD^+ is required for glycolysis. Another function of cytoplasmic GPDH is to provide precursors for phospholipids, since glycerolphosphate can be converted to phosphatic acid. It should be mentioned that the brain has no glycerokinase and therefore cannot make glycerolphosphate from glycerol. Mitochondrial glycerophosphate dehydrogenase (E.C.1.1.99.5) is not under hormonal control in the brain (de Vellis and Inglish, 1968) and in the ensuing discussion GPDH refers only to the cytoplasmic enzyme.

The concentration of glycerophosphate dehydrogenase in the rat brain is controlled by glucocorticoids. Figure 2 shows that following hypophysectomy or adrenalectomy of adult rats GPDH activity decreased to about 35% of control after 3 weeks (de Vellis and Inglish, 1968). Hypophysectomy of 20-day-old rats stopped the developmental increase of GPDH. In both instances, several other enzymes and brain protein content remained unchanged indicating that cortisol regulates GPDH specifically. Injection of cortisol to adrenalectomized rats, and ACTH (or cortisol) to hypophysectomized rats restored GPDH level to normal. As one might expect from the above results, thyroidectomy and gonadectomy of adult rats had no effect on GPDH concentration. Although not all tissues have yet been tested, the induction appears to be brain specific. GPDH has been purified from rat brain, characterized and injected into rabbits to obtain GPDH antisera. A given amount of GPDH antibody inactivates an equal amount of GPDH activity from control and induced animals (or glial cultures), indicating that GPDH is identical in the two preparations. It can be concluded that enzyme activity represents enzyme concentration and that cortisol increases the amount of enzyme rather than modifies the catalytic properties of GPDH (Mc Ginnis and de Vellis, 1973). The action of cortisol in the adult rat indicates that the differentiated brain is capable of metabolic adaptation, a fact largely unnoticed until recently (McIlwain, 1971).

Regulation of Glycerophosphate Dehydrogenase in the Developing Rat Brain

In order to facilitate the interpretation of our studies on GPDH development, it is worthwhile to summarize briefly the critical steps in the induction of GPDH by cortisol. The evidence for these regulatory mechanisms will be discussed later with the presentation of our studies of cultured cells. Both *in vivo* and *in vitro*, the presence of cortisol is required for the induction of GPDH and its maintenance. This phenomenon is dose-dependent. After entry of the hormone into the cell by diffusion, cortisol binds to a receptor protein (cytoplasmic receptor) and apparently the complex is translocated to the nucleus where it binds to an acceptor site (McEwen and de Vellis, unpublished results). Inhibition of nuclear uptake and binding of the hormone results in a correlative inhibition of the induction, indicating that binding of cortisol in the nucleus is a prerequisite for enzyme induction. Nuclear binding of the hormone occurs rapidly in a matter of minutes and precedes the requirement for *de novo* synthesis of RNA and protein specific to GPDH. Unlike the catecholamine induction of glial LDH, GPDH induction by cortisol is not mediated by cyclic AMP. Consequently, the concentration of GPDH at any age may depend on at least four factors: (1) the availability and concentration of cortisol, (2) receptor activity and nuclear binding of the hormone, (3) RNA synthesis and (4) protein synthesis.

Glial proliferation in the rat brain occurs mainly during the first 12 postnatal days. It is not known whether the development of GPDH is limited by any factors other than the appearance of glial cells and their growth. Among the factors cited above, hormone availability can be tested most easily. Cerebrum, brain stem and cerebellum were the brain regions studied. Daily injection of cortisol between the 3rd and 7th postnatal day did not increase GPDH level in the cerebrum and brain stem, but did cause a 2.4-fold increase in the cerebellum (Table 1). Daily administration of cortisol between 7 and 11 days of age increased GPDH activity in brain stem and cerebellum, but not in the cerebrum (Table 2). The brain stem showed a higher response than cerebellum. The same regional differences were observed when cortisol was injected for longer periods, up to 18 days of age (Table 3). No differences were noted between males and females.

The adult level of GPDH is reached at about 35 days of age (fig. 3, and de Vellis _et al_., 1967). Animals were injected with cortisol daily from day 7 to 16 or 41 days of age and all were sacrificed at 42 days of age (Table 4). The level of GPDH in treated and control animals at 42 days was identical. Cortisol injection in adults had no effect (Table 4). These results show that cortisol causes a premature appearance of GPDH in cerebellum and brain stem, i.e., the developmental curve of GPDH is shifted but its final level is not altered (fig. 3). The effect of administration of cortisol can be explained by the fact that cortisol levels in the blood are low. Indeed, the pituitary-adrenal axis is almost non-functional between the 4th and 10th postnatal day; after the 10th postnatal day, glucocorticoid secretion increases (Haltmeyer _et al_., 1966; Levine and Mullins, 1966). This was further tested by administration of ACTH from 7 to 10 days of age. Like cortisol, ACTH raised the level of GPDH in the brain stem but not in the cerebrum (de Vellis and Inglish, 1973). On the other hand, estradiol, which stimulates lipid accumulation in the developing rat brain (Casper _et al_., 1967) and accelerates functional brain maturation and myelination (Curry and Heim, 1966), had no effect on the development of GPDH (de Vellis and Inglish, 1973). Estradiol and several other hormones do not regulate GPDH in RGC_6 cells (de Vellis *et al.*, 1971b). These results indicate that during development and in adults cortisol is the hormone which specifically regulates GPDH. Furthermore, the potentiality for transcription of GPDH develops in the brain stem and cerebellum long before its actual synthesis. It is tempting to speculate that cortisol receptors and "nuclear competence" develops much earlier than the availability of cortisol. The factors which influence glial cells to become sensitive to cortisol remain unknown.

The lack of response in the cerebrum is more difficult to explain. It is known that glial cells appear later in cerebrum than in the brain stem. However, the cerebellum is also quite immature and yet responds to administration of cortisol. The activity present during the first 12 to 14 days after birth may represent a basal activity of GPDH which is not regulated by cortisol. Glial cells *in vitro* have a basal activity; and *in vivo*, hypophysectomized and adrenalectomized animals retain about 30% of the original activity several weeks after surgery (fig. 2). The cortisol regulated activity of GPDH may develop in the cerebrum after 15 days of age when the pituitary-adrenal axis is fully active. Culture of explants of prenatal rat cerebrum can be induced by cortisol (Breen, Col and de Vellis, unpublished data), thus invalidating the latter hypothesis.

The role of the other factors mentioned at the beginning of this section cannot be easily ascertained because of the difficulty of obtaining intact pure glial cells. A regional study of the concentration of cortisol receptors in glial cells during development is essential to fully understand the observed regional differences. Another approach is to use clonal cultures of glial cells which are a model system allowing quantitative biochemical measurements and also hopefully reflecting some of the activity of glial cells *in vivo*.

Induction of GPDH by Cortisol in Vitro

Recently, Breen, Cole and de Vellis (unpublished data) showed that GPDH can be induced in cultured explants (organotypic cultures) of several brain regions. However, our studies on the mechanisms of enzyme induction have been carried out using a clonal astrocytoma cell line, in order to take advantage of cell homogeneity.

The hormonal specificity of GPDH induction established *in vivo* was further confirmed in RGC_6 cells. Thyroid hormones, insulin, growth hormone, estradiol, testosterone, progesterone and catecholamines cannot induce GPDH. Furthermore, cortisol induces GPDH in cells maintained in serum free medium (de Vellis *et al.*, 1971b). Therefore, *in vivo* as *in vitro*, the presence of a glucocorticoid appears to be the only hormonal requirement for GPDH induction.

The basal activity of GPDH in some subclones of RGC_6 cells is shown in Table 5. It is worth noting that all clones were found to have a normal diploid karyotype. The inducibility of GPDH at 24 hr. does not correlate with basal activity, indicating that basal and induced activities are under separate control. A time course of the induction is shown in figure 4. A new steady state, usually 12 to 18 times higher than the basal level, is reached 5 days after addition of cortisol. The effect of cortisol concentration on GPDH induction is shown in figure 5. Saturation is reached at 10^{-7}M. Dexamethasone induces and saturates at lower concentrations. The corticosterone dose-response curve is similar to that of cortisol. Studies with these three hormones labeled with ^{3}H showed that there was an immediate nuclear uptake and retention of the hormone added to the culture medium (McEwen and de Vellis, unpublished data). In a variety of experimental conditions, GPDH induction correlated with nuclear binding of the hormone suggesting an action of glucocorticoids at the nuclear, hence transcriptional level. This conclusion is in agreement with the inhibitory effect of actinomycin D. Inhibitors of protein synthesis, like puromycin, acetoxycycloheximide and cycloheximide, inhibit GPDH induction, indicating that *de novo* protein synthesis is required (de Vellis *et al.*, 1971b). A further discussion of nuclear events will be presented below.

As I shall present later, unlike LDH, GPDH is not inducible by dibutyryl cyclic AMP (Table 10). This is in agreement with the fact that cortisol does not cause a rise in cyclic AMP in RGC_6 cells (Table 11). The addition of both norepinephrine and cortisol gives a GPDH induction identical to that obtained with cortisol alone, suggesting that cyclic AMP does not even have a secondary effect on GPDH induction.

Age-Dependent Changes in the Induction of Glycerophosphate Dehydrogenase in a Rat Glial Cell Line

S-100 protein accumulation in RGC_6 cells starts only after cultures have reached confluency (Benda *et al.*, 1968; Pfeiffer *et al.*, 1970). Unlike S-100 protein accumulation, GPDH induction was observed in cultures during logarithmic growth as well as in the stationary phase. In the original C_6 clone, little variation in inducibility of GPDH was observed with age of the culture (de Vellis and Inglish, 1969; de Vellis *et al.*, 1971a). However, clones 11 D and 2 B, which display good inductions, induced GPDH maximally 8 to 10 days after passage (fig. 6 and Table 6) confirming the observations of Davidson and Benda (1970) who used a subclone of C_6. Inducibility is very low in proliferating cells and in old cells (Table 6). Actually, inducibility is often nil one day after passage (fig. 6).

The reduced inducibility of GPDH in rapidly dividing cells (generation time 20 hours) and in old cells could be due to a reduction in the overall rate of synthesis of RNA and/or protein, or to a decrease in the nuclear uptake and binding of the hormone into the nucleus (or a combination of these factors) as compared to early stationary phase cells. Incorporation of uridine-2-^{14}C into RNA was highest in the old cells. There was little difference at the other two ages (Table 7). Incorporation of leucine-1-^{14}C into proteins decreased with age. However, this decrease may be more apparent than real since there was a corresponding reduction in the labeling of the free pool (Table 8). The third parameter, nuclear retention of cortisol, did vary with the age of the culture (Table 9). Nuclear retention was maximum at 10 days of age when inducibility is maximum. The reduction in inducibility observed in proliferating and old cells correlates with the reduction in nuclear retention of cortisol.

The results obtained with clonal glial cell cultures suggest that a lower hormonal receptor activity is responsible for the reduced inducibility of GPDH in proliferating and old cells. This conclusion points out the importance of studying the regulation of the cortisol receptor of glial cells *in vivo* during development and aging. Such studies might explain the observed regional differences in induction of GPDH during early postnatal development.

Effect of Catecholamines on Cyclic AMP and Lactic Dehydrogenase in a Rat Glial Cell Line

Lactic dehydrogenase (LDH) (E.C.1.1.1.27) is inducible by catecholamines but not by cortisol and several other hormones in RGC_6 cells (de Vellis and Inglish, 1969; de Vellis *et al.*, 1971b). The question arose as to whether cyclic AMP would induce LDH since many effects of catecholamines are known to be mediated by cyclic AMP. When dibutyryl cyclic AMP was used at concentrations up to 10^{-4}M, it had no effect on LDH. This result was rather surprising since dibutyryl cyclic AMP is thought to penetrate cells fairly well. Actually, RGC_6 cells and many other cells are not very permeable to this compound, though more permeable than to cyclic AMP. Higher millimolar concentrations induced LDH maximally (de Vellis, 1971) (Table 10). De Vellis and Brooker (1972) showed that cyclic AMP mediates the action of catecholamines on LDH.

The time course of LDH induction is shown in figure 7. After a lag of approximately 4 hours, there is a rapid rise in LDH activity which reaches a plateau after 20 hours. Preceding the rise in LDH is a large transient rise in the intracellular level of cyclic AMP. The correlation between cyclic AMP levels in cells and LDH induction can be seen in figure 8, which shows dose-response curves obtained with epinephrine and isoproterenol. At 3 x 10^{-9}M, isoproterenol causes a 3-fold increase in cyclic AMP and induces LDH half maximally. At 3 x 10^{-8}M isoproterenol causes a 30-fold increase in cyclic AMP and a full induction of LDH. Epinephrine is less potent than isoproterenol and requires a 10-fold increase in concentration to show the same effects. These results agree with well known physiological effects of these compounds in other tissues. Several compounds which may increase cyclic AMP levels in brain tissues (for review see Robinson *et al.*, 1971) were tested (Table 11). Tyramine, dopamine, histamine and adenosine have no effect on cyclic AMP level and LDH activity. Epinine, octopamine and phenylephrine, which approximately triple cyclic AMP concentration, induce LDH half maximally. These results are in agreement with those of Gilman and Niremberg (1971), who observed that dopamine, histamine and adenosine had no effect on cyclic AMP level of RGC_6 cells. However, a human astrocytoma cell line, 1181N1, was found to be responsive to histamine and adenosine

(Clark and Perkins, 1971, 1972). Finally, propranolol, a β-blocker, inhibits the rise in cyclic AMP and LDH induction whereas dibenzyline, an α-blocker, affects neither cyclic AMP nor LDH (Table 12), indicating that the effect of catecholamines is mediated by a β-receptor. The evidence for cyclic AMP as mediator of the catecholamine induction of LDH is: (1) only the compounds which cause a rise in intracellular concentration of cyclic AMP induce LDH, (2) the rise in cyclic AMP precedes LDH induction, (3) cyclic AMP and dibutyryl cyclic AMP mimic the action of the active hormones, and (4) compounds which block the rise in cyclic AMP inhibit the induction.

LDH induction appears to require *de novo* synthesis of protein and RNA since addition of actinomycin D, acetoxycycloheximide or puromycin with the hormone results in complete inhibition of the induction (de Vellis *et al.*, 1971b). The periods during which RNA synthesis and protein synthesis are required are shown at the bottom of figure 7. Time zero represents the time of addition of norepinephrine. Actinomycin D was added at several points between 0 and 6 hours. Total blockage of LDH induction occurred when actinomycin D was added at times up to 30 minutes; at later times the inhibition decreased, disappearing completely at 2.5 hours. However, addition of acetoxycycloheximide, an inhibitor of protein synthesis, inhibited totally the induction when added at 5 hours. The requirement for protein synthesis parallels the rise in LDH activity. To find out the period during which cyclic AMP is required (fig. 7) the following experiment was performed. The medium containing norepinephrine was removed at various times and replaced by fresh medium containing propranolol. This procedure decreased the intracellular concentration of cyclic AMP to basal level in a few minutes. LDH was assayed at 24 hours. When the propranolol wash out procedure was done after 2.5 hours, LDH induction was maximal, but at earlier times there was inhibition of the induction, suggesting that an elevated level of cyclic AMP is only necessary during the first 2.5 hours, i.e., during the *de novo* RNA synthesis period and not during the period of protein synthesis. Therefore, it appears that the magnitude of the LDH induction depends not only on the magnitude of the rise in cyclic AMP but also its duration. In other words, a transient rise in cyclic AMP of very short duration would not result in LDH induction.

The isoenzymes of LDH present in RGC_6 cells are V (MMM), IV and III. The induction by catecholamines shifts this pattern further toward V so that the increase in activity is the result of accumulation of more M subunits preferentially synthesized over the H type (Yu and de Vellis, 1973).

It has not been established yet that the effects of catecholamines on human and rat glial tumor cell lines represent function of normal glial cells _in vivo_. However, it is tempting to speculate that such functions as induction of S-100 protein and of GPDH represent specialized properties of nervous tissue which have been retained by cultured tumor cells. LDH induction has only been observed in neural cell cultures and, therefore, may be specific to nervous tissue. Until its physiological significance can be fully assessed, LDH induction represents a model system to study the role of cyclic AMP in enzymic differentiation. Our data indicate that cyclic AMP affects the transcription of LDH while in the liver, the site of action of cyclic AMP on enzyme induction may be at the level of translation (Wicks, 1971; Chuah and Oliver, 1971). Enzyme levels in the pineal gland are also regulated by cyclic AMP (Klein _et al_., 1970).

Differential Sensitivity of GPDH and LDH Inductions to Inhibitors of RNA Synthesis

Roeder and Rutter (1969, 1970) showed that three types of RNA polymerases may be separated from rat liver and sea urchin embryo nuclei on the basis of chromatographic properties and sensitivity to ions. RNA polymerase I is localized in the nucleolus and is responsible for the synthesis of ribosomal RNA. RNA polymerases II and III are situated in the nucleoplasm and synthesize giant nuclear heterogeneous RNA (Zylber and Penman, 1971). In isolated nuclei of RGC_6 cells, we showed the presence of three RNA polymerases (de Vellis and Inglish, 1972), using the method of Zylber and Penman (1971). The existence of specific inhibitors of the RNA polymerases made it possible to ask which polymerase(s) synthesizes the RNA required for induction of GPDH and LDH. RNA polymerase II is specifically inhibited by α-amanitin while the other two enzymes are not affected even at very high concentrations (Lindell _et al_., 1970). A low level of actinomycin D (0.04 µg/ml) inhibits ribosomal RNA synthesis but not giant nuclear heterogeneous RNA (Penman *et al.*, 1968).

GPDH induction is inhibited by α-amanitin whereas LDH induction is totally insensitive (Table 13). Inhibition of ribosomal RNA synthesis reduced GPDH but not LDH induction. This leaves RNA polymerase III to synthesize RNA necessary for LDH induction. That RNA is required for LDH induction is indicated not only by the inhibitory effect of actinomycin D added at 1 μg/ml but also by cordycepin, an inhibitor of mRNA synthesis (Penman *et al.*, 1970). Ethidium bromide, an inhibitor of mitochondrial RNA synthesis (Zylber *et al.*, 1969) had no effect on GPDH or LDH induction. The sensitivity of GPDH induction to low levels of actinomycin D suggests that either GPDH induction requires *de novo* rRNA synthesis in addition to mRNA synthesis or that the genes coding for GPDH, like those of rRNA, have a high affinity for actinomycin D.

The interpretation of results obtained with inhibitors of RNA and protein synthesis depends on their presumed specificity of action. Therefore, several important parameters of the two inductions were studied. Inhibitors had no effect on the nuclear uptake and retention of ^{3}H-cortisol, a prerequisite for the induction of GPDH. Inhibitors did not prevent the rise in cyclic AMP caused by addition of catecholamines. The effect of inhibitors on incorporation of leucine -1-^{14}C and uridine -^{14}C correlated with their presumed action. In conclusion, our results suggest that *de novo* RNA synthesis for GPDH is transcribed by RNA polymerase II and that for LDH by RNA polymerase III (de Vellis and Inglish, 1972). The RNAs may be transcribed from the structural or regulatory genes of these two enzymes. At the present time, it is not possible to distinguish between these two alternatives.

If indeed different genes are transcribed by different RNA polymerases, it implies that a change in the activity of one of the RNA polymerases will affect the rate of transcription of only some of the active genes. Thus, differential effect and specificity of action can be achieved by stimuli affecting RNA polymerases during development and aging.

Summary

RGC_6 cells provide us with a unique opportunity to study in the same cell type the mechanisms of action of glucocorticoids and catecholamines on enzyme induction. The observed differences in the mode of action of these two hormones are interesting, but much remains to be investigated. It is not known where glucocorticoids bind in cell nuclei nor what is the sequence of events in the nucleus which finally results in increased enzyme concentration in the cells. The model of Jacob and Monod (Jacob, 1966) for enzyme induction in bacteria has not been proven for the induction of enzymes by hormones in mammalian cells. Becuase of this, Tomkins, *et al.* (1969) proposed a model which postulates that cortisol induces enzymes by decreasing the rate of degradation of mRNA although direct evidence for this scheme is still lacking.

The loss of inducibility of GPDH in somatic cell hybrids (RGC_6-3T3 cells) (Davidson and Benda, 1970) and growth of cells in medium containing bromodeoxyuridine (Lyons and de Vellis, unpublished data) shows that GPDH induction shares many of the general characteristics of differentiated functions. These are usually extinguished by hybridization between a differentiated cell and a cell line lacking the parameter studied and also when cells are grown in bromodeoxyuridine.

Cyclic AMP as an inducer allows the cell to be responsive to all the stimuli which can activate its adenylcyclase. Changes in adenylcyclase-receptor sensitivity have been shown to occur in several tissues during development. This provides a mean for acquisition or loss of functions during development and aging. How does cyclic AMP induce enzymes? Does it bind to a cyclic AMP receptor protein as in bacteria (De Crombrugghe *et al.*, 1971) or does it activate a protein kinase? In the latter case, how is specificity achieved? Is it by phosphorylation of a histone or an acidic protein? The diversity of nuclear acidic proteins could provide specificity in activation of genes. The causal relationship between all these possible events has not yet been established in mammalian cells.

The sensitivity of glial adenylcyclase to one or even perhaps several neurotransmitters provide a mechanism to coordinate glial metabolism to that of neurons. Not only is enzyme induction affected by cyclic AMP but also the permeability of cultured glial cells is modified by catecholamine and cyclic AMP (Shinwari and de Vellis, 1972). Opler and Makman (1972) have also reported that glycogenolysis in these cells is increased by catecholamines.

The mechanisms which I have described give us some insight into enzymic differentiation and metabolic adaptation in the brain. It may be important to find out if these regulatory mechanisms change with aging.

Acknowledgements

This research was supported by Contract AT(04-1) Gen-12 from the Atomic Energy Commission and by United States Public Health Service grants HD-04612 and HD-05615.

References

Benda, P., Lightbody, L., Sato, G., Levine, L. and Sweet, W. (1968). Science 161, 370.

Brooker, G. (1970). Analyt. Chem. 42, 1108.

Burch, H.B., Lowry, O.H., Kuhlman, A.M., Skerjance, J., Diamant, E.J., Lowry, S.R. and Von Dippe, P. (1963). J. Biol. Chem. 238, 2267.

Casper, R., Vernadakis, A. and Timiras, P.S. (1967). Brain Res. 5, 523.

Chuah, C.C. and Oliver, I.T. (1971). Biochem. 10, 2990.

Clark, R.B. and Perkins, J.P. (1971). Proc. Nat. Acad. Sci. 68, 2757.

Clark, R.B. and Perkins, J.P. (1972). Fed. Proc. 31, 513.

Curry, J.J. and Heim, L.M. (1966). Nature 209, 915.

Davidson, R.L. and Benda, P. (1970). Proc. Nat. Acad. Sci. 67, 1870.

De Crombrugghe, B., Chen, B., Gottesman, M. and Pastan, I. (1971). Nature 230, 37.

de Vellis, J. (1970). In "Cell Differentiation" (O.A. Schjeide and J. de Vellis, eds.), pp. 284-321, Van Nostrand Reinhold, New York.

de Vellis, J. (1971). In "Contributions of clonal systems to neurobiology" Neurosci. Res. Bull. (in press).

de Vellis, J. and Brooker, G. (1972). Fed. Proc. 31, 513.

de Vellis, J. and Brooker, G. (1973). In "Tissue Culture of the Nervous System" (G. Sato, ed.), Vol. I, Plenum Press, New York (in press).

de Vellis, J. and Clemente, C.D. (1970). In "Cell Differentiation" (O.A. Schjeide and J. de Vellis, eds.), pp. 529-574, Van Nostrand Reinhold, New York.

de Vellis, J. and Inglish, D. (1968). J. Neurochem. 15, 1061.

de Vellis, J. and Inglish, D. (1969). 2nd Intern. Meet. Soc. Neurochem., Milan, Italy (R. Paoletti, B. Fumagalli and C. Galli, eds.),Tamburini Editore, Milan.

de Vellis, J. and Inglish, D. (1972). In Vitro 7, 247.

de Vellis, J. and Inglish, D. (1973). In "Progress in Brain Research" (D. Ford, ed.), Elsevier, Amsterdam (in press).

de Vellis, J., Schjeide, O.A. and Clemente, C.D. (1967). J. Neurochem. 14, 499.

de Vellis, J., Inglish, D. and Galey, F. (1971a). In "Cellular Aspects of Growth and Differentiation in Nervous Tissue" (D. Pease, ed.), pp. 23-32, University of California Press, Berkeley and Los Angeles.

de Vellis, J., Inglish, D., Cole, R. and Molson, J. (1971b). In "Influence of Hormones on the Nervous System" (D. Ford, ed.), pp. 25-39, Karger, Basel.

Giacobini, E. (1964). In "Morphological and Biochemical Correlates of Neural Activity" (M. M. Cohen and R. S. Snider, eds.), pp. 15-38, Harper and Row, New York.

Gilman, A.G. and Niremberg, M. (1971). Proc. Nat. Acad. Sci. 68, 2165.

Haltmeyer, G.C., Denenberg, V.H., Thatcher, J. and Zarrow, M.X. (1966). Nature 212, 1371.

Herschman, H.R., Levine, L. and de Vellis, J. (1971). J. Neurochem. 18, 629.

Holliday, R. and Tarrant, G.M. (1972). Nature 238, 26.

Jacob, F. (1966). Science 152, 1470.

Klein, D.C., Berg, G.R. and Weller, J. (1970). Science 168, 979.

Levine, S. and Mullins, R.F. (1966). Science 152, 1585.

Lindell, T.J., Weinberg, F., Morris, P.W., Roeder, R.G., Rutter, W.J. (1970). Science 170, 447.

McCaman, R.E. and Robins, E. (1959). J. Neurochem. 5, 32.

McGinnis, J.F. and de Vellis, J. (1973). Fed. Proc. 32,604.

McEwen, B.S., Weiss, J.M. and Schwartz, L.S. (1970). Brain Res. 17, 471.

McIlwain, H. (1971). In "Essays in Biochemistry" (P.N. Campbell and F. Dickens, eds.), Vol. 7, pp. 145-158, Academic Press, London and New York.

Millichop, J.G. (1957). Proc. Soc. Exptl. Biol. Med. 96, 125.

Opler, L.A. and Makman, M.H. (1972). Biochem. Biophys. Res. Comm. 46, 1140.

Orgel, L.S. (1963). Proc. Nat. Acad. Sci. 49, 517.

Penman, S., Vesco, C. and Penman, M. (1968). J. Mol. Biol.

34, 49.
Penman, S., Rosbach, M. and Penman, M. (1970). Proc. Nat. Acad. Sci. 67, 1878.
Perez, V.J., Olney, J., Cicero, T.J., Moore, B.W. and Bahn, B.A. (1970). J. Neurochem. 17, 511.
Pfeiffer, S.E., Herschman, J.R., Lightbody, J. and Sato, G. (1970). J. Cell. Physiol. 75, 329.
Robinson, G.A., Butcher, R.W. and Sutherland, E.W. (1971). "Cyclic AMP", Academic Press, New York.
Roeder, R.G. and Rutter, W.J. (1969). Nature 224, 234.
Roeder, R.G. and Rutter, W.J. (1970). Proc. Nat. Acad. Sci. 65, 675.
Shinwari, M.A. and de Vellis, J. (1972). 3rd Meet. Amer. Soc. Neurochem., Seattle, p. 121.
Tomkins, G.M., Gelehrter, T.D., Granner, D., Martin, D., Samuels, H.H. and Thompson, E.B. (1969). Science 166, 1474.
Venter, C., Dixon, J.W., Maroko, P.R. and Kaplan, N.O. (1972). Proc. Nat. Acad. Sci. 69, 1141.
Wicks, W.D. (1971). J. Biol. Chem. 246, 217.
Yu, G. and de Vellis, J. (1973). Fourth Meet. Amer. Soc. Neurochem., Columbus, Ohio, p. 145.
Zylber, E.A. and Penman, S. (1971). Prod. Nat. Acad. Sci. 68, 2861.
Zylber, E.A., Vesco, C. and Penman, S. (1969). J. Mol. Biol. 44, 195.

TABLE 1

Effect of administration of cortisol from the 3rd to the 7th day of age on the activity of GPDH at 8 days in various brain regions.*

		GPDH (Units/mg protein)	
		S.A.	% Control
Cerebrum	Control (4)	11.2 ± 0.3	100.0 ± 2.3
Cerebrum	Cortisol (4)	11.8 ± 0.3	105.6 ± 3.0
Brain Stem	Control (4)	5.6 ± 0.3	100.0 ± 5.2
Brain Stem	Cortisol (4)	6.6 ± 0.6	117.0 ±10.7
Cerebellum	Control (4)	8.2 ± 0.4	100.0 ± 4.3
Cerebellum	Cortisol (4)	20.4 ± 2.0	248.2 ±23.8

*Cortisol (0.5 mg per 30 gm body weight) was injected daily from the 3rd to the 7th day after birth. Animals were killed on the 8th day. GPDH was assayed and specific activity (S.A.) determined as outlined in methods. Number of animals are indicated in parentheses. Data represent mean ± S.D.

TABLE 2

Effect of administration of cortisol from the 7th to the 11th day of age on the activity of GPDH at 12 days in various brain regions.*

Brain Region	Treatment	GPDH S.A. (% control)
Cerebrum	Control	100 ± 2.1
Cerebrum	Cortisol	103 ± 4.1
Brain Stem	Control	100 ± 1.5
Brain Stem	Cortisol	165 ± 5.0
Cerebellum	Control	100 ± 3.5
Cerebellum	Cortisol	140 ± 4.1

*Animals were injected daily from the 7th to the 10th day and killed on the 12th day. For other conditions see Table 1 and the methods.

TABLE 3

Effect of cortisol administration between 7 and 14 days and between 7 and 18 days of age on GPDH activity.*

	Injected	Killed	GPDH, S.A. (% Control)		
			Cerebrum	Brain Stem	Cerebellum
Expt. 1	7-14 d	15 d			
male (3)			114.2 ± 3.1	160.3 ± 0.0	--
female (3)			110.0 ± 1.0	158.6 ± 15.5	--
Expt. 2	7-18 d	19 d			
male (1)			125.0	152.4	137.3
female (4)			113.2 ± 5.6	140.9 ± 6.4	121.3 ± 9.1

*Rats (littermates) were injected subcutaneously at the nape of the neck for the age periods indicated with cortisol at a dose of 0.5 mg/30 gm body weight per day. Animals were sacrificed at the indicated ages. An equal number of controls was used. Results are expressed as mean ± S.D. Number of animals is in parentheses.

TABLE 4

Effect of cortisol administration between 7 and 16 days and between 7 and 41 days of age on GPDH activity at 42 days.

		GPDH, S.A. (% Control)		
Injected	Killed	Cerebrum	Brain Stem	Cerebellum
7- 16 d(4)	42 d	106.3 ± 2.0	102.7 ± 3.1	102.2 ± 4.3
7- 41 d(4)	42 d	99.4 ± 4.1	95.4 ± 5.1	97.1 ± 5.5
120-130 d(4)	131 d	102.1 ± 3.1	95.9 ± 4.1	104.1 ±49.0

For explanations see Table 3.

TABLE 5

Basal level and induction of GPDH in various subclones of RGC_6 cells.*

Clone	Control Units/mg protein	+ Cortisol % Control
C-6	50.8 ± 7.1 (15)	171.0 ± 9.8 (15)
G-10	9.50± 0.21 (3)	170.1 ± 8.6 (3)
9-F	17.2 ± 1.2 (4)	152.3 ± 11.5 (4)
11-D	52.0 ± 2.9 (3)	268.1 ± 35.5 (3)
9-E	65.4 ± 11.9 (4)	188.9 ± 5.8 (4)
2-B	51.0 ± 4.1 (6)	300.5 ± 15.4 (6)

*Cortisol succinate was added at a final concentration of 1.33 µg/ml of medium. Enzyme activity was measured 24 hrs later as described in the text.

TABLE 6

Cortisol induction of glycerol phosphate dehydrogenase in log phase, stationary phase and aging cultures of RGC_6 cells.*

Age (Days)	Treatment	GPDH (S.A.)	GPDH (% Control)
3	Control (4)	18.0 ± 1.0	100.0 ± 5.4
3	Cortisol (4)	31.4 ± 3.7	174.8 ± 20.3
10	Control (3)	49.3 ± 2.4	100.0 ± 4.8
10	Cortisol (3)	169.8 ± 12.6	344.1 ± 25.6
38	Control (5)	17.0 ± 1.8	100.0 ± 10.4
38	Cortisol (5)	38.6 ± 1.2	226.8 ± 6.8

*Cortisol was added at a final concentration of 0.2 µg/ml medium. Enzyme activity was measured 24 hrs. later as indicated in the methods.

TABLE 7

Incorporation of uridine - 2 - ^{14}C into RNA of log phase, stationary phase and aging cultures of RGC_6 cells.*

Age (Days)	RNA cpm/µg RNA	Free Pool cpm/µg RNA
4 (4)	772 ± 7	3371 ± 150
10 (4)	878 ± 26	3490 ± 270
32 (3)	1511 ± 107	3550 ± 220

*Cultures were pulsed for 1 hour with one µc of uridine - 2 - ^{14}C/3 ml of Ham's medium supplemented with 10% fetal calf serum.

TABLE 8

Incorporation of leucine - 1 - ^{14}C into proteins of log phase, stationary phase and aging cultures of RGC_6 cells.*

Age (Days)	Proteins cpm/mg protein	Free Pool cpm/mg protein
4 (4)	63823 ± 1116	14367 ± 685
16 (4)	51542 ± 1193	13174 ± 401
32 (4)	40516 ± 2978	8673 ± 481

*Cultures were pulsed for 1 hour with leucine - 1 - ^{14}C (0.5 μc/3 ml of Ham's F10 medium supplemented with 10% fetal calf serum).

TABLE 9

Nuclear retention of ^{3}H-cortisol in log phase (3 days), stationary phase (10 days), and aging cultures (32 days) of RGC_6 cells.*

	Age (Days)	Nuclei cpm/mg protein	% whole cell radioactivity recovered in nuclei
Expt. 1	10	48,480	15.6
	3	32,480	5.9
Expt. 2	10	58,500	22.1
	32	30,200	11.1

*Cells were incubated for 30 minutes in the presence of ^{3}H-cortisol (8 μc/ml of medium (2×10^{-7}M) at 37°C). Cells were washed 8 times with 0.9% NaCl, homogenized in 0.32 M sucrose containing 3 mM $MgCl_2$, 1 mM KH_2PO_4, and 0.25% triton X. Nuclei were isolated by the method of McEwen, *et al.* (1970) and the radioactivity extracted in a toluene liquid scintillation fluid.

TABLE 10

Effect of norepinephrine (NE), cortisol and dibutyryl cyclic AMP (DBcAMP) on GPDH and LDH inductions in RGC_6 cells.*

Treatment	GPDH Units/mg protein % control	LDH Units/mg protein % control
Control	100.0 ± 4.1	100.0 ± 5.0
DBcAMP, 10^{-4}M	90.1 ± 1.9	98.1 ± 5.8
DBcAMP, 5 x 10^{-4}M	100.1 ± 6.0	160.0 ± 3.8
DBcAMP, 10^{-3}M	103.4 ± 9.1	207.1 ± 13.5
NE, 10^{-6}M	100.1 ± 5.1	208.2 ± 10.6
Cortisol, 1.38x10^{-6}M	350.0 ± 30.1	108.1 ± 4.6
NE + Cortisol	345.1 ± 20.1	205.6 ± 8.1

*Compounds were added to the culture medium at the indicated final concentrations. GPDH and LDH were assayed at 24 hrs. Specific activity is expressed as per cent control ± S.D.

TABLE 11

Effect of catecholamines and other compounds on cyclic AMP level and LDH activity in RGC_6 cells.*

Treatment	Cyclic AMP pmoles/mg protein % control	LDH units/mg protein % control
Control	100	100
Tyramine, 3 x 10^{-5}M	90 ± 5	96 ± 3
Dopamine, 3 x 10^{-5}M	90 ± 6	98 ± 7
Histamine, 10^{-4}M	100 ± 8	101 ± 4
Adenosine, 1.25 x 10^{-4}M	100 ± 7	99 ± 3
Epinine, 3 x 10^{-5}M	400 ± 100	148 ± 11
Octopamine, 3 x 10^{-5}M	300 ± 80	141 ± 5
Phenylephrine, 3 x 10^{-5}M	320 ± 30	146 ± 5
Norepinephrine, 3 x 10^{-5}M	3500 ± 180	185 ± 9
Cortisol, 2.7 x 10^{-6}M	108 ± 10	110 ± 6

*All compounds were added to the culture medium at the final concentrations indicated above. Cyclic AMP was measured 45 min. later. LDH activity was determined at 24 hrs. in another set of cultures. Cyclic AMP was measured according to Brooker (1970). (From de Vellis and Brooker, 1973.)

TABLE 12

Effect of α- and β-blockers on the action of norepinephrine on RGC_6 cells.

Treatment[1]	Cyclic AMP pmoles/mg protein	LDH units/mg protein % control
Control	7 ± 3	100
NE	337 ± 32	213 ± 8
NE + propranolol	7 ± 2	117 ± 12
NE + dibenzyline	327 ± 95	225 ± 15

[1]All compounds were added to the culture medium at a final concentration of 3 x 10^{-5}M. Cyclic AMP was measured 45 min. later. LDH activity was determined at 24 hrs. in another set of cultures. The effects of epinine, octopamine and phenylephrine on cyclic AMP and LDH were similarly blocked by propranolol but not by dibenzyline (from de Vellis and Brooker, 1973).

TABLE 13

Effect of inhibitors of RNA synthesis on LDH and GPDH induction in RGC_6 cells.*

Treatment	GPDH units/mg protein % control	LDH units/mg protein % control
Control	100	100
Induced (NE + Cortisol)	350 ± 30	205 ± 20
α-Amanitin (10^{-5}M)	145 ± 11	210 ± 25
AMD**(0.05 μg/ml)	165 ± 5	207 ± 12
AMD**(1 μg/ml)	101 ± 6	98 ± 7
Cordycepin (2 x 10^{-4}M)	180 ± 8	145 ± 12
Ethidium bromide (1 μg/ml)	360 ± 1	213 ± 8

*Compounds were added to the culture medium at the final concentration indicated above. NE and cortisol were added as in Table 10. GPDH and LDH were assayed at 24 hrs.

**Actinomycin D

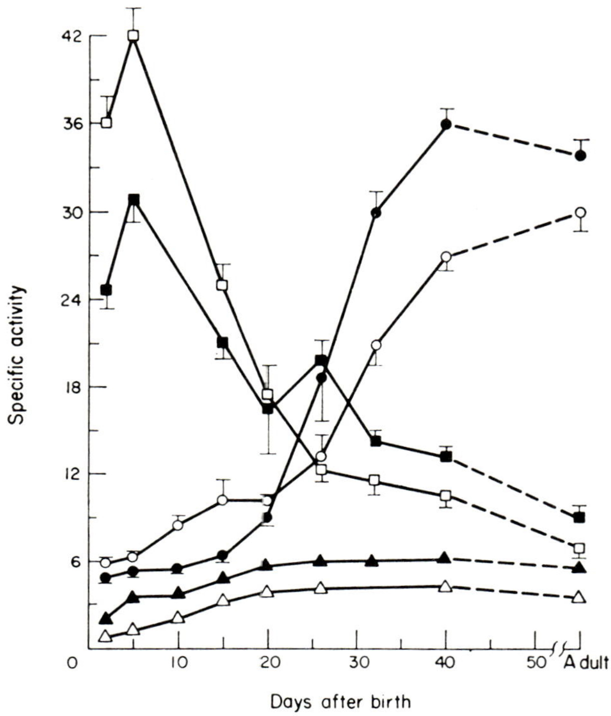

Fig. 1 Variation of the specific activities of glycerophosphate dehydrogenase (o), isocitrate dehydrogenase (□), and malate dehydrogeanse (1.1.1.40) (△) in the cerebrum (clear symbols) and in the brain stem (dark symbols) as a function of age. Each point represents the mean of at least three experiments comprising three to six animals each. Vertical bars represent S.D. depicted as either + or - S.D. values for malate dehydrogenase (1.1.1.40) are smaller than the size of the symbols. (From de Vellis *et al.*, 1967.)

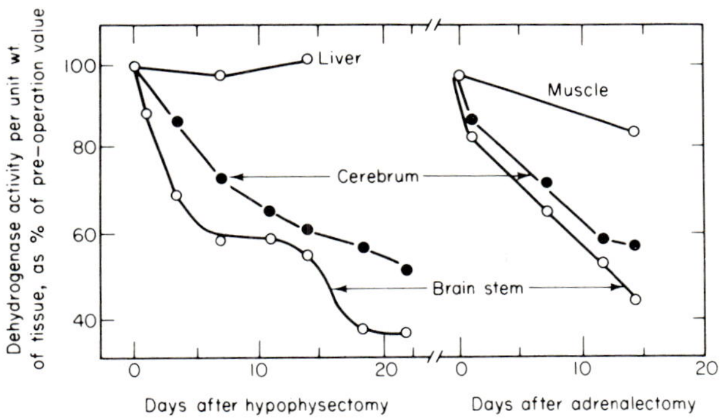

Fig. 2 Glycerophosphate dehydrogenase activities in tissues of adult rats following hyphophysectomy or adrenalectomy. (From de Vellis and Inglish, 1968.)

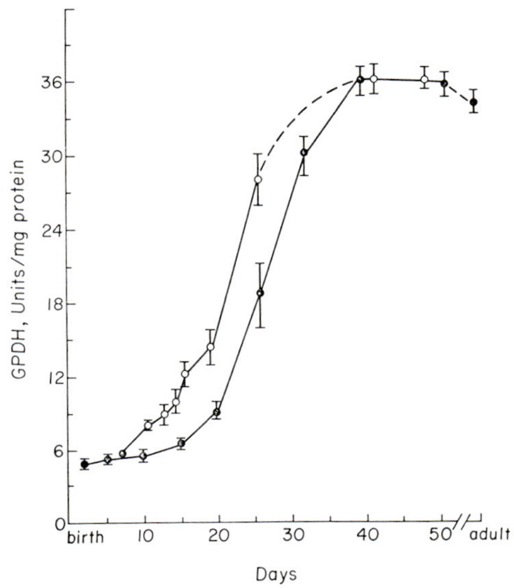

Fig. 3 Effect of cortisol on the developmental curve of GPDH in the brain stem. Rats were injected daily with 0.5 mg cortisol/30 gm body weight from 7 days of age until the day before sacrifice. Dark symbols represent control animals. Clear symbols represent animals injected with cortisol. Each point represents at least the mean of 3 animals ± S.D. (From de Vellis and Inglish, 1973.)

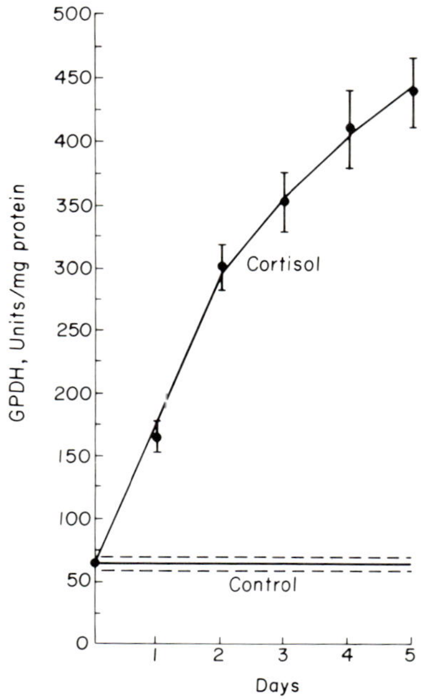

Fig. 4 Time course of GPDH induction by cortisol in RGC_6 cells. Cortisol was added at a final concentration of 5×10^{-7}M. The culture medium was changed every 24 hr. (From de Vellis and Inglish, 1973.)

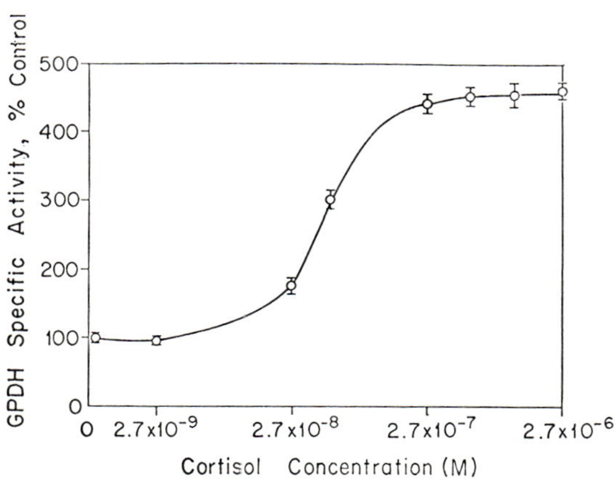

Fig. 5 Effect of cortisol concentration on GPDH induction in RGC_6 cells. Cortisol was dissolved in ethanol and added in 10 µl. Cultures were assayed 24 hrs. later. (From de Vellis and Inglish, 1973.)

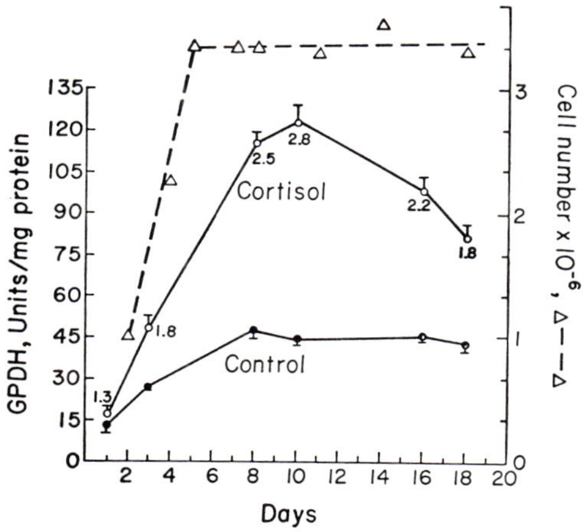

Fig. 6 Inducibility of GPDH in RGC_6 cell cultures at various ages. Dark circles represent the basal level of GPDH in 11D subclone. Clear circles represent the level of GPDH after a 24 hr. induction by cortisol and the number near each symbol represents the increase over basal level. The average cell numbers in each flask is given by triangles. Each point represents the average of 4 cultures ± S.D. (de Vellis and Inglish, 1973.)

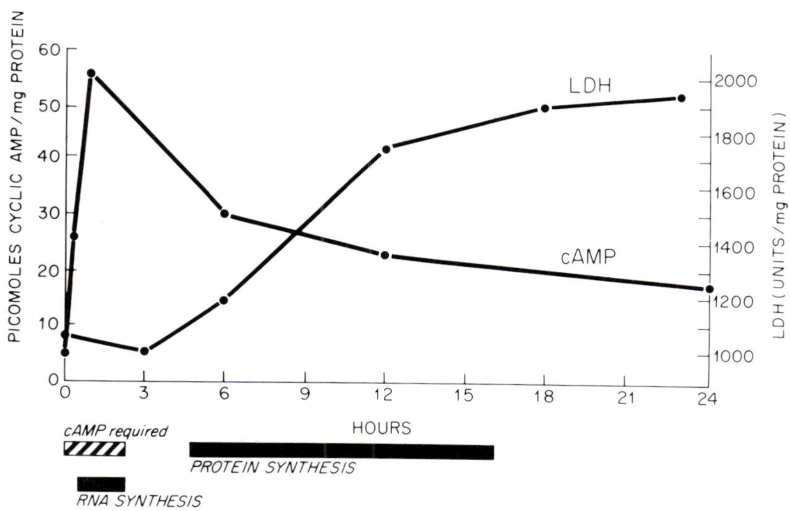

Fig. 7 Time course of cyclic AMP level and LDH induction in RGC_6 cells following the addition of norepinephrine to the culture medium. Norepinephrine was added at a final concentration of 3×10^{-5}M. Cyclic AMP was measured using high pressure anion exchange liquid chromatography (de Vellis and Brooker, 1973).

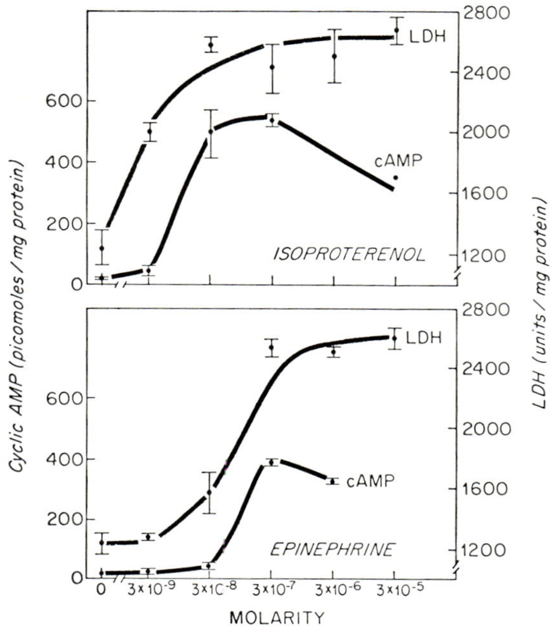

Fig. 8 Effect of isoproterenol and epinephrine concentration on cyclic AMP and LDH levels of RGC_6 cells. Cyclic AMP was measured 45 min. after addition to the culture medium of the indicated concentrations of epinephrine and isoproterenol. LDH activity was measured at 24 hr. on another set of cultures (de Vellis and Brooker, 1973).

MONOAMINE METABOLISM IN THE AGING MALE MOUSE

Caleb E. Finch, Ph.D.

The Laboratory of Neurobiology
The Ethel Percy Andrus Gerontology Center
University of Southern California
Los Angeles, California 90007

A fundamental and unresolved problem in experimental gerontology concerns the location of the pacemakers of aging. The term pacemaker connotes mechanisms which regulate the chronology and order of sequence of physiological changes which occur normally during the course of aging in mammals (Finch, 1972a; 1973). At present, there is no consensus as to whether pacemakers of aging reside within each cell in the organism (<u>intrinsic cellular pacemakers</u>) or whether there is a limited cell population (e.g., in the reticuloendothelial or neuroendocrine systems) which direct the course of aging in other cells and tissues throughout the body by humoral factors or neural signals (<u>extrinsic cellular pacemakers</u>) (Finch, 1969; 1971; 1972a,b; Finch *et al.*, 1969a,b). A type of intrinsic pacemaker was discovered by Hayflick (1970), who observed that euploid fibroblast cell strains from the adult human lung have a finite lifespan in culture of about 40 generations. The limited lifespan of these cells is governed by a pacemaker within those cells and does not simply result from exhaustion of a nutrient in the medium, since cells from early ("young") and late ("old") cultures when grown together conform to their separate schedules of aging. However, this particular model of aging is probably not general because no normally dividing cell line exhausts its capability for proliferation (e.g., the exfoliating epithelial populations of the intestinal mucosa (Lesher, 1966)) during the lifespan (reviewed in Finch, 1969). Furthermore, even the most ardent cell culture enthusiast must concede that the media to which cells may become adapted in culture cannot exactly recreate the complete environment of ionic, macromolecular factors and heterotypic cell to cell interactions of the intact organism. It is indeed remarkable that so many differentiated cell characters can persist in long-term cell cultures (Davidson, 1964).

In the past decade, examples have also accumulated which show that at least some cellular changes in the whole mammal during aging result from humoral or neural factors extrinsic to that cell. An illustration that an age-related change in liver cell function may result from changes outside the liver was observed by the author in a study of the regulation of liver tyrosine aminotransferase (TAT) (Finch *et al.*, 1969a). The enzyme TAT was discovered to be induced very rapidly in the livers of young mice during exposure to cold (Finch *et al.*, 1969b); the increase was linear, extrapolating back to the moment of exposure to cold. However, in mice older than 24 months, there was a long delay of up to 2 hours before the increase in the enzyme could be observed (Finch *et al.*, 1969a); after the end of the delay, the rate of increase was approximately that observed in younger mice. This observation poses the question: were the liver cells in old mice unable to respond rapidly to the stimuli (presumably hormonal or neural) which increased the level of the enzyme so rapidly in the young mice; or contrarily, did the age-related event outside of the liver cell originate in the system of neural and endocrine control influencing the liver's production of TAT? This question was resolved, in part, by our findings that the injection of hormones known to act directly on the liver (insulin and corticosterone) could induce the enzyme with the same kinetics in both young and old mice. This experiment, therefore, shows that old liver cells can respond as rapidly as young liver cells given the appropriate stimulus and implicates external or extrahepatic factors as the basis for the age change. Although the locus (presumably neuroendocrine) of age change in the system of tyrosine aminotransferase regulation remains unidentified, the general conclusion of our study is consistent with a number of other studies of the liver: that basic cellular function is maintained throughout the lifespan when the appropriate stimulus is present, e.g. the observations on a different hepatic enzyme system of Adelman (1970). The exemplary studies of Makinodan and colleagues of age-related changes in cellular immune mechanisms also clearly demonstrate distinctions between intrinsic and extrinsic factors of cellular aging (reviewed in Makinodan et al., 1971; Price and Makinodan, 1972a,b).

Extra-cellular or hormonal factors of aging have been chemically characterized in only two different vertebrates: the Pacific salmon (Onchorhynchus sp.) and the post-menopausal human female. In the case of the Pacific salmon, both sexes of five species die of adrenal corticosteroid toxicosis after their first spawning (Robertson et al., 1961; see Finch et al., 1969a and Finch, 1971 for further discussion of this remarkable phenomena). The agents mediating widespread and selective changes in cell function during aging in the Pacific salmon have been identified as predominantly hydrocortisone but also cortisone, whose levels in the blood increase five-fold. This hormonal change is undoubtably not a normal phenomenon of aging in mammals; on the contrary the meager existing evidence about adrenal cortical function in mammals suggests some decline in corticosteroid production. Among the few humoral changes which have been characterized in humans and other mammals during aging is the loss of ovarian steroid production after menopause; a decline to 5-10% of the normal monthly output of estrogens is typical (Pincus, 1956; McBride, 1957; Paulsen et al., 1958). Concomitantly, pituitary gonadotrophin production increases (Pincus, 1956; Paulsen et al., 1958). There is a great deal of information indicating that many of the changes in cells of female mammals during aging are secondary to the great post-menopausal reduction in ovarian steroids of females. Effect of the 90-95% loss of ovarian steroids is observed in many tissues. Although particularly prominant in cells of those tissues such as the uterus and the vagina, which are estrogen dependent, changes in the vasculature may also be direct consequences of the loss of ovarian steroids (Kurland and Freedburg, 1960; Malinov et al., 1964).

In cases of the postreproductive ovary, it appears that this organ is capable still of producing normal amounts of steroids. In a fascinating experiment, Clemens, et al. (1969) were able to re-initiate ovarian cycles in post-estrous (23 months old) female rats by briefly electrically stimulating the pre-optic region of the hypothalamus, a brain region known to control the regulation of the cycles of gonadotrophic hormones which, in turn, drive the ovarian cycles. This experiment indicates how age-related changes in a relatively minute region of the body (the pre-optic nuclei) may serve as a pacemaker of aging (in this case, for the ovary) with consequences to cells throughout the body. It thus appears that the age-related changes in many cell types result from the response of those cells to factors in their environment as is particularly demonstrated for estrogen-dependent tissues, and among others, the pituitary (Pecile *et al.*, 1966) and prostrate (Mainwaring, 1968), it may be said that at least some changes are not directly by pacemakers of aging intrinsic to those cells. Because of the indications that hormones may figure prominently in at least some cellular aging changes of vertebrates *in vivo*, we have begun to investigate the seats of control of endocrine and autonomic functions in the brain. This program has also been undertaken to eventually test the hypothesis that the brain may contain pacemakers for some events of aging.

There is, at present, relatively little information of how aging affects cell function in the mammalian brain. One of the most important and unresolved questions in this area concerns the relation of vascular disease to cellular function in the brain during aging. Many studies have shown an extremely high frequency of advanced vascular disease in the human brain after the age of 70 years (Mathur *et al.*, 1963; Flora *et al.*, 1968). It is therefore difficult, at present, to establish that changes in brain cell function during aging are independent of the reduced blood supply or the cellular death resulting from a compromised blood supply. To distinguish changes of aging associated with disease from "normal" aging changes, we have introduced the terms *pathogeric* and *eugeric* (Finch, 1972a) which connote changes which are secondary to the diseases of aging (pathogeric) in distinction to those whose immediate cause is not a pathologic change (eugeric). A common example of pathogeric changes may be found in the loss of recent memory following vascular lesions (stroke) involving the hippocampus. It seems plausible that early studies reporting massive widespread neuronal loss in the brain of humans and other mammals during aging (reviewed in Finch, 1969) included brain tissue which was badly damaged by arteriosclerosis and other vascular lesions. It appears from recent studies of Brody (see this symposium) that neuronal loss during aging in humans may not be as generalized as previously considered and, in fact, may be restricted to a few areas of the brain: at least some nuclei do not lose detectible numbers of cells (e.g., the inferior olive). At the present time it is safe to say that most neurons in the brain survive from birth to old age and that massive loss of neurons and brain tissue during aging is not a usual consequence of aging.

Because of the extremely widespread incidence of vascular disease during aging in most human populations, it may be useful to employ smaller, shorter-lived mammals in order to distinguish eugeric changes in brain function from those consequent to cerebral vascular lesions. Surprisingly little appears to be known about spontaneous cerebral vascular disease in mammals. A recent publication by Nanda and Getty (1971) shows definite, widespread and progressive thickening of the intima in the aging pig. Corresponding changes were not found in the aging dog, whose cerebral arterial walls developed fibrosis; intimal thickenings were restricted to "pial and intracerebral" branches. Some rodent strains may provide valuable experimental models because massive cerebral vascular disease probably is relatively rare in this order of mammals. Unfortunately, information about spontaneous cerebral vascular disease appears to be very scanty; the few studies known to me have not verified the extent of the phenomena.

A fascinating study of spontaneous arteriosclerosis in several strains of inbred rats by B.C. Wexler and collaborators has revealed that the virgin Sprague-Dawley rats of both sexes have minimum lesions in coronary and carotid vessels and none in cerebral arteries. However, if rats of either sex are bred repeatedly, severe arteriosclerosis develops by one year of age in the coronary and great vessels; in rats whose carotid arteries showed extensive arteriosclerosis, lesions in the intracranial arteries were detected (Wexler, 1964a,b). However, there was "no evidence of cerebral damage" in even the most arteriosclerotic rats (Wexler and True, 1963). Unilateral experimental ligation of the carotid arteries in rats was found to produce cerebral edema in virgin and arteriosclerotic breeds of both sexes; however, gross cerebral ischemia, hemorrhage or necrosis was "scant, occurring only on an erratic basis in all groups..." (Wexler and Sardoff, 1970). In contrast, bilateral carotid ligation produced grossly visible hemorrhage and necrosis (Wexler, 1970). It thus appears that Sprague-Dawley rats are relatively protected from analogues of cerebral vascular disease and stroke in humans.

A few other reports of cerebral vascular lesions may be cited. A small subpopulation (perhaps 34/700) of mice of four strains (VM,C57, RIII, and MM; both sexes included) 279 days or older were observed by Fraser (1967) to show bilateral ectopic calcification in the thalamus. A microscopic examination of the brains of 2-3-year-old A/J mice revealed a high incidence of "substantial calcium deposits, apparently in the small blood vessels of the hypothalamus". Senescence in this strain is particularly interesting because of an apparent absence of pathological changes (tumors, arteriosclerosis, renal lesions); the primary cause of death in old age was anorexia, perhaps resulting from vascular lesions in the hypothalamic centers controlling appetite (Coburn _et al_., 1971). The apparently divergent findings of Wexler (1963; 1964a,b; 1970), Fraser (1967), and Coburn (1971), as described above, may have resulted from differences in diet, genetic factors, behavioral history and age at examination. In any case, the incidence of spontaneous cerebral vascular disease is a major issue in studying brain function during aging and, at present, must be resolved by each investigator.

We have employed the mouse as a model system for aging changes in human brain. The C57 BL/6J mouse has a lifespan of approximately 30 months and, within that span of 30 months, manifests many of the same physiological changes observed in humans over a much longer period of time. If one divides the maximum lifespan into fractions, many of the same developmental and physiological changes then are placed in corresponding fractions of the lifespan of short and long-lived mammals (Finch, 1971). Therefore, it is not unreasonable to use a short-lived rodent as a model of aging for some aspects of the human brain. For example, the events of reproductive senescence in the female, the accumulation of comparable amounts of aging pigment and the loss of autonomic control mechanisms such as thermoregulation (Finch _et al_., 1969a) do occur in corresponding fractions of lifespan of both mice and men. There may, of course, be aging phenomonen which are more purely time-dependent which could not be recognized in the lifespan of a 30-month-old mouse.

In 1966, the author founded a colony of C57 BL/6J male mice while a graduate student at the Rockefeller University. Because of rigorously maintained conditions of husbandry, this colony has an unusual profile of health during most of adult lifespan; the incidence of diseases before the age of 24 months is less than 1% (Finch et al., 1969a; Finch and Foster, 1973). After 24 months, a solid tumor of the liver and often the spleen appears with increasing incidence, the reticulum cell sarcoma (which is a common cause of death in this strain (Finch et al., 1969a; Dunn, 1954). Because of the prevalence of tumors and other pathological conditions in mice of the older age groups, Finch, et al. (1969a) and Finch and Foster (1973) developed criteria for identifying aging mice without major pathological lesions; only such mice are used in our experiments. This necessitates the culling of over 50% of the older mice, but we are sure that the mice used in our experiments provide a representative sample of mice of that age group without interference from advanced stages of a terminal disease. Although exhaustive studies of the brain have not been undertaken, limited sampling of mice of various ages have not revealed major cerebral histopathology. This supposition is born out by the uniformity of the data obtained on samples of old mice (e.g., no age difference in coefficient of variation, Tables 1 and 3).

We have initiated our study of cellular mechanisms in the aging mammalian brain by an investigation of neurotransmitter metabolism in C57 BL/6J male mice. The rationale for this investigation was provided by a variety of evidence that important changes in autonomic functions occur during aging. In a previous investigation, for example, we showed that senescent mice (28 months) became deficient in their ability to maintain body temperature during brief exposures to cold (Finch et al., 1969a). It is well known that monoamines are of fundamental importance to thermal regulatory mechanisms. Indications that aging may affect monoamine metabolism was deduced from other studies. (I) The selective effect of age on the phases of the human sleep cycle (stage IV and REM sleep are reduced (Feinberg, 1969); regulation of sleep is dependent on monoaminergic mechanisms). (II) The re-initiation of ovarian cycles after pre-optic stimulation (Clemens et al., 1969) which, together with experiments showing that reserpine arrested estrous can be overcome by pre-optic stimulation, implies monoaminergic transmitter alteration. (III) Finally, findings in idiopathic Parkinson's disease in which catecholamine levels were reduced in specific brain regions

(Hornykiewicz, 1965). Unfortunately, these studies did not include age-related controls of the same age group without Parkinson's disease. Thus it remained possible that the changes in monoamines were, at least to some extent, an aspect of the normal process of aging.

We first measured monoamine levels in the brains of aging mice. Mice of two age groups were employed in all of these experiments; mature mice, which have achieved the maximum body weight under our conditions of husbandry (these mice are aged 10-12 months) and senescent mice (aged 28-30 months) at the average maximum lifespan in the colony (Finch *et al.*, 1969a). These mice, as mentioned earlier, are selected for the absence of gross pathological conditions shown at necropsy. Microscale adaptations of standard fluorometric assays (Shellenberger and Gordon, 1971) permitted measurement of monoamines in individual mouse brains and brain regions. No significant changes of whole brain dopamine, norepinephrine and serotonin were found in mice up to the age of 30 months. However, measurements on specific regions revealed dopamine is decreased by about 25% in the striate body of aging mice. These changes, summarized in Table 1 below, while not as extreme as those observed in human Parkinsonism, emphasize the importance of age as a variable in the analysis of Parkinson's disease. No other brain region examined showed a change of catecholamine level during aging; norepinephrine in cerebellum, brain stem and hypothalamus. Other observations in neurotransmitter metabolites are summarized in Table 2, in which the paucity of data is perhaps the most outstanding feature. Because of the extraordinary spectrum of differentiated cell types in the brain (represented, for instance, in the great amount of unique DNA sequence transcription, which is 3-4 times greater in the brain than in visceral organs such as liver and kidney (Hahn and Laird, 1971; Brown and Church, 1971), studies of neurotransmitter metabolites of small brain regions will probably prove to be far more illuminating than those of whole brains or large regions, such as hindbrain or brain stem).

We then studied the metabolism of catecholamines as a function of age. Our study of catecholamine metabolism utilized two precursors of catecholamines which were injected peripherally (i.p.). Tritiated tyrosine and tritiated L-Dopa were found to enter the blood from the peritoneal cavity (the locus of injection) with the same efficiency in both mature and senescent mice (Finch, 1973). However, the conversion of these precursors to catecholamines in the aging mouse brain was significantly reduced in at least four regions: hypothalamus, striatum, brain stem and cerebellum. We observed that the total level of radioactivity in these brain regions after i.p. injection of tyrosine or L-Dopa was the same in both age groups (Table 3); this implies that the tritiated precursor passed with some efficiency in the blood and into the brain tissue in both age groups. Subsequently, however, the amount of precursor converted to dopamine or norepinephrine was much reduced in the senescent mice (Table 3). Our data may be summarized by the statistical statements that the conversion of precursors was 1.6±.1 times greater in mature than in senescent mice. Because decreased efficiency of conversion to catecholamines was observed with both L-tyrosine and L-Dopa as precursors, it is possible that there is a block in the enzymatic step converting L-Dopa to dopamine. However, the activity of Dopa decarboxylase (the enzyme which converts L-Dopa to dopamine) did not reveal any age-related change in the hypothalamus or striatum of mice (Finch, 1973). The precise location of the aging change therefore cannot be ascertained at the present time: reasonable alternatives include the reduced transport of precursors from the blood into the pre-synaptic regions where monoamines are synthesized, faulty uptake of dopamine by the pre-synaptic catecholamine storage vesicles, or a shift towards increased catabolism.

The possibility of increased catabolism of monoamines is supported by observations of elevated monoamine oxidase activity during aging. These data, summarized in Table 4, are the best established of the enzymatic changes observed in neurotransmitter metabolism. As found in a previous review of enzyme activities during aging, the changes observed are selective; most enzyme activities, as measured in cell-free homogenates, are not affected greatly during aging (Finch, 1972b).

Current studies in our laboratory are focusing on the uptake of monoamines and their precursors *in vitro*. Our findings to date are summarized in Table 5. At physiological concentrations of tyrosine, only a very slight difference is observed in the uptake of tyrosine by the hypothalamus. Nonetheless, the difference is consistently observed. Further experiments will reveal if age-related decrease in transport efficiency in the brain is a general finding.

Other studies indicate that the turnover of catecholamines labeled with ^{3}H-L-Dopa as a precursor (i.p. injected) is significantly slower in senescent mice as compared with mature mice: this is demonstrated for hypothalamic norepinephrine and striatal dopamine (Finch, 1973). Because extra-neuronal pools of L-Dopa are known to accumulate after L-Dopa administration, we cannot be sure at this time that we are measuring the turnover of stores of catecholamines in the pre-synaptic vesicles. However, it is reasonable to conclude that there is a fundamental alteration of brain catecholamine metabolism during aging which includes reduced neuronal catecholamine metabolism in at least two brain regions. We are pursuing these studies further with the use of tyrosine as a precursor and measurement of the endogenous tyrosine stores in the brain regions as a function of aging. It is not practical at the present time to measure L-Dopa pools in the minute brain regions of aging mice, available only in small numbers.

The above changes in monoamine metabolism in the brain could have much significance to a variety of neuroendocrine functions which are known to be affected by aging. In particular, the observations of Clemens, *et al.* (1969) that the preoptic region of the hypothalamus may be stimulated to initiate normal estrous cycles in senescent female rats supports our hypothesis of altered monoamine metabolism during aging. Our data on the slowed turnover of hypothalamic norepinephrine and striated dopamine directly support this conclusion. Importantly, for the human extra-pyramidal diseases, including Parkinson's disease, there appears to be a loss of dopamine as we have shown above in the striate body. It is therefore reasonable to hypothesize that the age-related increase in Parkinson's and other extra-pyramidal syndromes results from the tendency of the mammalian brain to lose striatal dopamine stores during aging. This possibility remains to be documented in normal human brain tissue of the ages corresponding to Parkinson's disease. A recent study indicating 40-50% reductions of norepinephrine in normal human hindbrain during aging (Robinson *et al.*, 1972) is supportive of the hypothesis; dopamine was not measured in the study. The hypothesis that a lowered threshold for extra-pyramidal diseases results from the declining stores of neurotransmitters during aging is also supported by a study showing that phenothiazine-induced extra-pyramidal symptoms can be induced much more easily in older, normal patients (Ayd, 1961). (Phenothiazines produce a loss of brain dopamine under certain conditions (O'Keefe et al., 1970).) Additionally, irreversible choreiform facial movements are induced much more readily by phenothiazine in older aged patients (Siede and Müller, 1967). Therefore, the interesting possibility arises that Parkinson's and other common extra-pyramidal conditions of aging constitute extreme developments of normal changes of aging (Finch, 1973).

The evidence of Walker and Boas-Walker (1973) that the sensitivity of adenyl cyclase to catecholamines is reduced in the caudate, cerebellum, cortex and hippocampus of senescent rats provides a mechanism for amplifying the consequences of reduced catecholamine levels and turnover in the brain during aging. It appears, moreover, given the sensitivity of catecholamine metabolism to hormones (e.g., thyroid (Emlen et al., 1972) and adrenal and gonadal steroids (Prange et al., 1970; Anton-Tay et al., 1970)) and the role of monoaminergic systems in the control of the hypophyseal-pituitary axes (McCann, 1970), that a regulatory cascade, involving interplay between changing levels of hormone production by endocrine glands and hormone sensitive sites in the brain, which serve as pacemakers and/or relays for outgoing neural/humoral signals could be a basis for many endocrine and autonomic changes of age. A hypothetical fragment of such a regulatory cascade may be constructed from the following observations; cessation of cyclic ovarian function during reproductive senescence does not appear to be the result of primary ovarian failure, since, upon transplantation to a young host, an old ovary will show normal estrous cycles and can yield fertile ova (Talbert and Krohn, 1966); rather, the defect appears to be central, based on the reactivation of estrous by pre-optic stimulation in senescent rats (Clemens et al., 1969). The cessation of ovarian steroidogenesis during reproductive senescence in rodents and humans "derepresses" the output of pituitary gonadotrophins (this is probably not deleterious in itself) and, in addition, reduces the output of growth hormone which has an estrogen-dependent burst in the human female on normal first awakening in the morning (Frantz and Rabkin, 1965). In turn, the reduced output of growth hormone could alter the metabolism of

GH-sensitive tissues, such as liver and thyroid, whose metabolic products, in turn, influence brain cell function.

It is therefore possible that the "rigid" intrinsic models of aging involving generalized pacemakers of aging in each cell throughout the body or the restriction of pacemakers to certain cell groups (neuroendocrine or reticuloendothelial cell subpopulations) are both incomplete, if aging involves regulatory cascades in which changes in cell function at discrete loci, perhaps "originating" at the time of maturation, result in a chain of events. Thus, the preconditions for the next stage of aging may be regulated by pacemakers specific to that physiological stage of aging and different from those of preceding or succeeding stages.

The concept that aging in mammals is best analyzed as part of a developmental continuum, in which the mechanisms for the transition from one stage to the next are established during preceding stages, may be relevent to progeria. Some evidence for this may be drawn from the various types of progeria (Hutchinson-Guilford's (affecting children) and Werner's (affecting adults) syndromes) in which truncated or arrested growth or development nearly always precedes the manifestation of premature aging (Epstein *et al.*, 1966; Reichel *et al.*, 1971; Villee *et al.*, 1969). It is therefore possible that some aspects of post-maturational aging are linked in a non-trivial way to cessation of growth or other previous developmental triggers.

In summary, the brain, by its over-riding influence on cell activities throughout the body, doubtless has a major influence on aging of somatic cells. The role of monoaminergic mechanisms in aging is undefined, but the involvement of the monoamines systems in neuroendocrine output and, in turn, the sensitivity of monoamine metabolism to hormonal state influences (gonad, adrenal, thyroid) provide possibilities of regulatory cascades involving cell activities throughout the body. The observations on altered catecholamine metabolism in C57 BL/6J male mouse brains described in the present paper, may therefore reflect one "time frame" on a sequence of events begun at a much earlier stage of development.

REFERENCES

Adelman, R.C. (1970). J. Biol. Chem. 245, 1032.
Anton-Tay, F., Anton, S.M. and Wurtman, R.J. (1970). Neuroendocrinol. 6, 265.
Ayd, F.J. (1961). J. Am. Med. Assoc. 175, 1054.
Brown, I.R. and Church, R.B. (1971). Biochem. Biophys. Res. Commun. 42, 850.
Burton, K. (1962). Biochem. J. 62, 315.
Clemens, J.A., Amenomori, Y., Jenkins, T. and Meites, J. (1969). Proc. Soc. Exp. Biol. Med. 132, 561.
Coburn, A.F., Grenard, R.M. and Rivera, S.M. (1971). John Hopkins Med. J. 128, 169.
Davidson, E.H. (1964). Advan. Genet. 12, 143.
Dunn, T.B. (1954). J. Nat. Cancer Inst. 14, 1281.
Emlen, W., Segal, D.S. and Mondell, A.J. (1972). Science 175, 79.
Epstein, C.J., Martin, G.M., Schultz, A.L. and Motulsky, A.G. (1966). Medicine 45, 177.
Feinburg, I. (1969). In "Sleep Physiology and Pathology" (A. Kales, ed.), Ch. 3, J. B. Lippincott, Philadelphia, Pa.
Finch, C.E. (1969). "Cellular Activities During Ageing in Mammals", Ph.D. Dissertation, The Rockefeller University New York, pub. 1972 by MSS Information Systems, 655 Madison Ave., N.Y.C.
Finch, C.E. (1971). In "Animal Models for Biomedical Research, IV", pp. 47-67, National Academy of Sciences, U.S.A.
Finch, C.E. (1972a). In "Proceedings of the 1st Inter-National Conference on Cell Differentiation", Nice, 1971, (R. Harris and D. Viza, eds.) pp. 259-262, Munksgaard.
Finch, C.E. (1972b). Exp. Gerontol. 7, 53.
Finch, C.E. (1973). Brain Res. 52, (in press).
Finch, C.E. and Foster, J.R. (1973). Lab. Animal Sci. (in press).
Finch, C.E., Foster, J.R., and Mirsky, A.E. (1969a). J. Gen. Physiol. 54, 690.
Finch, C.E., Huberman, H.S. and Mirsky, A.E. (1969b). J. Gen. Physiol. 54, 675.
Flora, G.C., Baker, A.O., Loewenson, R.B. and Klassen, A.C. (1968). Circulation 38, 859.
Foldes, I., Csotortok, L. and Beregi, E. (1965). Gerontol.

Clin. 7, 92.
Frantz, A.G. and Rabkin, M.T. (1965). J. Clin. Endocrinol. 25, 1470.
Fraser, H.J. (1967). J. Pathol. Bacteriol. 96, 220.
Freedman, L.S. (1972). Nature 236, 310.
Gey, K.F., Burkard, F. and Pletcher, A. (1965). Gerontologia 11, 1.
Gottfries, C.G., Gottfries, I., Johansson, B., Olson, R., Persson, T., Roos, B.T. and Sjostrom, R. (1971). Neuropharmacol. 10, 665.
Hahn, W.E. and Laird, C.D. (1971). Science 173, 158.
Hayflick, L. (1970). Exp. Gerontol. 5, 291.
Hollander, J. and Barrows, C.F. (1968). J. Gerontol. 23, 174.
Hornykiewicz, O. (1965). In "Proceedings of the 2nd Symposium of the Parkinson's Disease Information and Research Center" (E. Costa, L. J. Côté and M. D. Yahr, eds.), Raven Press.
Kurland, G.S. and Freedberg, A.S. (1960). Circulation 22, 464.
Lesher, S. (1966). In "Radiation and Ageing" (P.G. Lindop and G. Sacher, eds.), pp. 183-188, Taylor and Francis, London.
Mainwaring, W.I.P. (1968). Gerontologia 14, 133.
Makinodan, T., Perkins, E.H. and Chen, M.G. (1971). Advan. Gerontol. Res. 3, 171.
Malinov, M.R., Moguilevsky, J.A., and Gerschenson, L.(1964). Circulation Res. 14, 364.
Mathur, K.S., Kashyap, S.K. and Kumar, V. (1963). Circulation 27, 929.
McBride, J.M. (1957). J. Clin. Endocrinol. Metab. 17, 1440.
McCann, S.M. (1970). In "The Hypothalamus" (L. Martini, M. Motta and F. Fraschini, eds.) pp. 277-292, Academic Press, New York.
McGeer, E.G., Fibiger, H.C., McGeer, P.L. and Wickson, V. (1971). Exp. Gerontol. 6, 391.
Nanda, B.S. and Getty, R. (1971). Exp. Gerontol. 6, 453.
O'Keefe, R., Sharman, D.F. and Vogt, M. (1970). Brit. J. Pharmacol. 38, 287.
Paulsen, C.A., Leach, R.B., Sandberg, H., Sheinfeld, S. and Maddock, W.O. (1958). J. Am. Geriat. Soc. 6, 803.
Pecile, A., Miller, E., and Falconi, G. (1966). Arch. Int. Pharm. 159, 434.
Pincus, G. (1956). In "Hormones and Ageing" (E.T. Engle

and G. Pincus, eds.) pp. 1-19, Academic Press, New York.
Prange, A.J., Meek, J.L. and Lipton, M.A. (1970). Life Sciences 9, 901.
Price, G.B. and Makinodan, T. (1972a). J. Immunol. 108,403.
Price, G.B. and Makinodan, T. (1972b). J. Immunol. 108,413.
Reichel, W.R., Garcia-Bunnel, R. and DiIallo, J. (1971). J. Am. Geriat. Soc. 19, 369.
Robinson, D.S., Nies, A., Davis, J.N., Bunney, W.E., Davis, J.M., Coburn, R.W., Bowrne, H.R., Shaw, D.M. and Coppen, A.J. (1972).Lancet i, 290.
Robertson, O.H., Krupp. M.A., Thomas, S.F., Favour, C.B., Hane, S. and Wexler, C. (1961). Gen. Comp. Endocrinol. 1, 473.
Samorajski, T., Rolsten, C. and Ordy, J.M. (1971). J. Gerontol. 26, 168.
Shellenberger, M.K. and Gordon, J.H. (1971). Anal. Biochem. 39, 356.
Siede, H. and Müller, H.F. (1967). J. Am. Geriat. Soc. 15, 517.
Talbert, B.G. and Krohn, P.L. (1966). J. Reprod. Fertility 11, 399.
Villee, D.B., Nichols, G. and Talbot, N.B. (1969). Pediatrics 43, 207.
Vulcana, T. and Timiras, P.S. (1969). In "Proceedings of 8th International Congress of Gerontology", p. 24., pub. by Fed. Am. Soc. for Exp. Biol.
Walker, J.P. and Boas-Walker, J. (1973). Brain Res. (in press).
Wexler, B.C. (1964a). Circulation Res. 14, 32.
Wexler, B.C. (1964b). Atherosclerosis Res. 4, 57.
Wexler, B.C. (1970). Stroke 1, 112.
Wexler, B.C. and True, C.W. (1963). Circulation Res. 12, 659.
Wexler, B.C. and Sardoff, J. (1970). Stroke 1, 38.
Wurtman, R.J. (1964). J. Clin. Endocrinol. Metab. 24, 299.

TABLE 1

Mouse Brain Catecholamine Levels During Aging

	ng/mg DNA X ± SEM[1]	Change[2]
Dopamine		
Striatum: mature[3]	3,215 ± 130	
senescent	2,515 ± 80	-22% ($p < .001$)
Norepinephrine		
Brain Stem: mature	750 ± 35	0
senescent	770 ± 30	
Cerebellum: mature	37 ± 3	0
senescent	34 ± 2	
Hypothalamus: mature	210 ± 14	0
senescent	236 ± 9	

[1]mean ± standard error of mean
[2]mature-senescent/mature x 100
[3]mature mice, aged 10-12 months; senescent mice, aged 28-30 months.

Catecholamines were measured in brain regions of individual mice by the procedure of Shellenberger and Gordon (1971). Catecholamine levels are expressed per mg DNA (Burton modification of the diphenylamine reaction, Burton, 1962) which permits an accurate measure of cellularity without incurring undesirable delays in freezing the tissue which are inherent in most weighing procedures. A minimum of 19 mice were sampled from each group. (Methods in Finch, 1973.)

Table 2

Aging and Monoamine Metabolite Levels

Substance	Change	Tissue	Ages	Subject	Sex	Author
Catecholamines						
dopamine	-20%	striatum	12 vs 28 mo.	C57BL/6J mouse	male	Finch, 1973
norepinephrine	0	whole brain	12 vs 28 mo.	C57BL/6J mouse	male	Finch, 1973
	0	cerebellum	12 vs 28 mo.	C57BL/6J mouse	male	Finch, 1973
	0	hypothalamus	12 vs 28 mo.	C57BL/6J mouse	male	Finch, 1973
	0	brain stem	12 vs 28 mo.	C57BL/6J mouse	male	Finch, 1973
	-5-10%	whole brain	9 vs 28 mo.	C57BL/10 mouse	male	Samorajski *et al.*, 1971
	-40-50%	hindbrain	25 vs 65+yr.	human	both	Robinson *et al.*, 1972
homovanillic acid	+100%	CSF	(18-29) vs (70-79) yr.	human	both	Gottfries *et al.*, 1971
Indolealkylamines						
serotonin	0	whole brain	12 vs 28 mo.	C57BL/6J mouse	male	Finch, 1973
	0	whole brain	15 vs 28 mo.	C57BL/10 mouse	male	Samorajski *et al.*, 1971
	0	hindbrain	25 vs 65+yr.	human	both	Robinson *et al.*, 1972
5-hydroxy indole acetic acid	0	hindbrain	25 vs 65+yr.	human	both	Robinson *et al.*, 1972
	+30%	hindbrain	65 vs 70 yr.	human	both	Robinson *et al.*, 1972
	+35%	CSF	(18-19) vs (70-79) yr.	human	both	Gottfries *et al.*, 1971
	-50%	urine (24 hr.)	(20-40) vs $>$80 yr.	human	both	Foldes *et al.*, 1965

TABLE 3

Conversion of Tyrosine and L-Dopa to Catecholamines in the Aging Mouse Hypothalamus

	Mature/Senescent
L-^{3}H-tyrosine precursor	
total acid soluble (^{3}H/mg DNA)[1]	1.03
dopamine (^{3}H-DA/mg DNA)[1]	1.22
norepinephrine (^{3}H-NE/mg DNA)[1]	2.37
cumulative ratio, 2 regions[2]	
dopamine	1.26 ± .06
norepinephrine	1.79 ± .19
L-^{3}H-Dopa precursor	
total acid soluble (^{3}H/mg DNA)[1]	1.05
dopamine (^{3}H-DA/mg DNA)[1]	1.46
norepinephrine (^{3}H-NE/mg DNA)[1]	1.77
cumulative ratio, 4 regions[3]	
dopamine	1.63 ± .14
norepinephrine	1.69 ± .07

[1]average, two experiments
[2]hypothalamus and brain stem
[3]hypothalamus, cerebellum, brain stem and striatum

Mice were injected i.p. with L-^{3}H (3,5) tyrosine or L-^{3}H (4,5) Dopa and were killed after 45 minutes. Norepinephrine and dopamine were isolated after separation from precursors and methylated and oxidized metabolites by chromotography on Alumina and Dowex 50 (Na^{+}). For complete details, see Finch (1973).

Table 4

Aging and Enzymes of Neurotransmitter Metabolism[1]

Enzyme	Change	Tissue	Ages	Subject	Sex	Author
Catecholamines						
tyrosine hydroxylase	-35%	striatum	(4-15) vs (28-29) mo.	Wistar rats	male	McGeer *et al.*, 1971
	0	brain, excepting striatum and cerebellum	(4-15) vs (28-29) mo.	Wistar rats	male	McGeer *et al.*, 1971
Dopa decarboxylase	0	hypothalamus	12 vs 28 mo.	C57BL/6J mice	male	Finch, 1973
	0	striatum	12 vs 28 mo.	C57BL/6J mice	male	Finch, 1973
	0	heart	15 vs 24 mo.	albino rat	both	Gey *et al.*, 1965
dopamine B-hydroxylase	+20%	serum	(21-40) vs (41-60) yr.	human	both	Freedman, *et al.*, 1972
catecholamine O-methyl transferase	0	heart	12 vs 24 mo.	albino rat	female	Gey *et al.*, 1965
monoamine oxidase	+25%	heart	8 vs 24 mo.	albino rat	male	Gey *et al.*, 1965
	+250%	heart	8 vs 24 mo.	albino rat	female	Gey *et al.*, 1965
	+80%	hindbrain	45 vs 65 yr.	human	both	Robinson *et al.*, 1972
	+50%	serum	55 vs 65 yr.	human	both	Robinson *et al.*, 1972
Indolealkylamines						
hydroxyindole-O-methyl transferase	-20%	pineal	(40-55) vs (55-70) yr.	human	both	Wurtman *et al.*, 1964
Acetylcholine						
Choline-acetylase	0	cerebral cortex hypothalamus, cerebellum	12,14,20 mo.	Long-Evans rat	male	Vulcana and Timiras, 1969
	-15%	spinal cord	2,12,20 mo.	Long-Evans rat	male	Vulcana and Timiras, 1969
acetyl-cholinesterase	0	whole brain	10 vs 29 mo.	Wistar rat	female	Hollander and Barrows, 1968
	0	whole brain	4 vs 28 mo.	C57BL/6J mice	both	Hollander and Barrows, 1968
	0	whole brain	9 vs 28 mo.	C57BL/10 mice	male	Samorajski *et al.*, 1971

[1]The citations in the above table are restricted to post-maturational ages and do not include comparisons of earlier ages or studies of animals in which body weight is the only parameter specifying age.

TABLE 5

Uptake of ^{3}H-L-Tyrosine into Hypothalamic Slices *In Vitro* in Mature and Senescent Mice[1] (CPM/mg Tissue Protein)

	Mature		Senescent	
Conditions	No. of Mice	CPM	No. of Mice	CPM
0° C/15 min.	6	98 ± 10	7	82 ± 11
37° C/15 min.	6	278 ± 33	6	266 ± 15
0° C/30 min.	6	115 ± 5	7	120 ± 12
37° C/30 min.	6	395 ± 15	6	366 ± 13

[1]0.25 mm slices of hypothalamus were incubated in pre-gased Krebs-Ringer phosphate buffer containing .015 μg (^{3}H) tyrosine/ml (52c/mM) under an atmosphere of 95% O_2 - 5% CO_2 in a Dubnoff metabolic shaker. The slices were washed at the end of incubation with ice-cold Krebs-Ringer phosphate and then homogenized in 0.25M PCA; protein was determined in the centrifugal pellet by the Lowry procedure.
Although differences between mature and senescent mice are consistent, they are not statistically significant.